NEVER LOSE YOUR VOICE AGAIN: The SECRET to Unlimited Vocal Health™ for Singers, Actors, and Speakers

By Katti Power

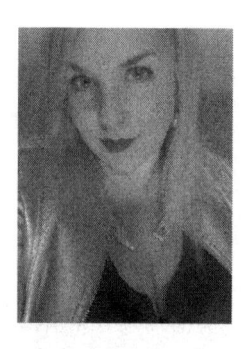

A FREE GIFT!

**As my thank you to you,
I'd love to share a free training called:**
*The SECRET To Never Losing
Your Voice Again*
which you can watch here:
www.singwithoutlimits.com/thesecret

Copyright 2021 Katti Power All right reserved. This book or parts thereof may not be reproduced in any form, stored in any retrieval system, or transmitted in any form by any means — electronic, mechanical, photocopy, recording, or otherwise — without prior written permission of the publisher, except as provided by United States of America copyright law. For permission requests, write to the publisher, at **kpower@kattipower.com**, or visit the author's website at **www.kattipower.com**

PREFACE

June 7, 1999. It's the first day of rehearsal. The six of us singers have three weeks in the United States to begin learning six shows before we fly to Nantes, France to board our brand-new cruise ship and sail it across the Atlantic, through the Panama Canal, and then across the Pacific, all the way to Tahiti. There, we'll spend the next nine months entertaining passengers on ten-day cruises in the Tahitian islands.

I was so excited. I love the ocean and boats of all kinds and had always wanted to see a whale, which I was convinced would happen during this contract. Plus, as someone who grew up in the suburbs of Chicago, and then went to school in NYC, I'd had my fair share of winter! I was thrilled to get to spend almost a year in a tropical paradise. I'd never even seen a cruise ship in person, much less been on one, and now I was about to make one my home! Much like my fascination with whales, I couldn't wrap my mind around how big the cruise ship would be, so I was eager to see it up close. It didn't disappoint!

Before heading to France to meet our cruise ship, the R3, we had to rehearse in Charlotte, NC for three weeks. We started by learning the "On Broadway" show, a revue with excerpts of major songs from musical theatre. There were three guys and three gals in our cast, and I was assigned the top soprano line/melody in all the songs. I was also the "belter" in the group. Not only did I sing the highest in all the group portions of our songs, I had the bulk of the big, belty solos, and I also sang the solos with the highest notes.

During those first three weeks of rehearsal, all the other cast members lost their voices except me. Because of that, and because of all my singing in the stratosphere and belting my face off, I earned the nickname, "Cords of Steel," from my fellow cast members and my music director. Most of the cast continued to experience voice loss periodically during our nine-month contract which was something I, the assigned vocal captain for our shows, had to anticipate and have a backup plan in place so we could continue with a show if someone had to call out because of voice loss or illness. This policy is pretty normal in the world of live performance; voice loss, after all, was something the industry expected to happen.

About halfway through my contract, I started noticing my voice sounding a little "husky." I brushed it off, justifying that I was really tired and probably spent too much time with my friends in the smoky crew bar.

I kept singing in the shows. Probably not my wisest move, as the problem started to worsen. I noticed I required considerably more air to sing than I usually did, and that no matter how hard I tried, certain notes just didn't seem to want to come out at all. There was a scene in our "Bandstand Boogie" show where I had to play this obnoxious, cartoon-y cheerleader and my voice for this role suddenly became very squeaky. I couldn't brush off the struggle anymore; something clearly wasn't right.

Then, one morning, I woke up to no voice at all.

Completely terrified, I decided to go to the ship doctor to get it checked out. He sent me to an ENT who did a scope of my vocal cords -- SUPER fun experience, by the way -- where I was informed I'd developed polyps. Polyps on your cords are fluid-filled lesions that prevent the cords from coming together all the way which causes voice loss or silent gaps in the vocal range.

I felt like I was in a nightmare that I couldn't wake myself from. The doctor recommended vocal rest so I could heal, but the only way I could go on vocal rest was to break my contract early and go home. Breaking my contract meant paying my replacement's way to Tahiti from North America and paying my own way home from Tahiti. Plus, as the vocal captain, it was my responsibility to train all new people on their vocals which meant adding rehearsals to my already demanding schedule and weakened voice.

My company was not thrilled with my news and wanted me to stay and finish out my contract. But staying required four more months of singing through this issue and the risk of permanent vocal damage. So, even though I was terrified of making a foolish choice, I decided to leave the ship to heal rather than jeopardize my budding career.

When I got home, I decided that while I rested my voice, I would do some research to figure out how I got myself into this crazy mess. I wanted to make sure I never had to deal with voice loss again. That research led to what I later formalized into my Unlimited Vocal Health™ System which I will share in this book.

I had no idea at the time that what I discovered on my own and put into practice was my own little SECRET. Voice loss prevention was unknown to the singing industry. I assumed I uncovered information everyone else already knew but that I somehow hadn't yet learned. However, once I started coaching singers, I was able to see that the steps I put together to form my vocal method weren't at all common knowledge. Singers often suffered like I had, without any method of prevention. I made the decision that everyone needed to learn what I had uncovered because of my own devastating experience with voice loss. I'm proud to report that not only have I never lost my voice again, but 100% of my clients over the past two decades haven't lost their voices either since doing this work with me.

And that is why, despite what medical professionals, vocal pedagogues, and other highly-degreed voice experts may say to the contrary, the evidence I've gained over two decades of work in this area has proven that voice loss ISN'T inevitable. It's preventable.

And I'm ready to stop keeping this preventability a SECRET.

TABLE OF CONTENTS

INTRODUCTION	1
PART I:	
FOUNDATION – VOCAL CORE POWER	8
1: EVERY BREATH YOU TAKE	9
2: SING OUT LOUD, SING OUT STRONG	21
3: COME TOGETHER RIGHT NOW OVER ME	36
4: PART I THE BULLSHIT BREAKDOWN	42
PART II:	
PLACEMENT – LIMITLESS POWER & RANGE	51
5: TOO LEGIT TO QUIT	52
6: SING OUT, LOUISE!	68
7: WISH I COULD BE PART OF THAT WORLD	79
8: PART II THE BULLSHIT BREAKDOWN	94
PART III:	
SHAPE – HIGH-POWERED HIGH NOTES	104
9: PUMP UP THE VOLUME, DANCE	105
10: WIDE OPEN SPACES	111
11: A CHANGE WOULD DO YOU GOOD	118
12: PART III THE BULLSHIT BREAKDOWN	125

PART IV:
CONSISTENCY – POWERFUL HABITS FOR CONSISTENT HEALTH 137
- 13: SILENCE SPEAKS A THOUSAND WORDS 138
- 14: YOU GOT THE RIGHT STUFF, BABY 150
- 15: PART IV THE BULLSHIT BREAKDOWN 162

CONCLUSION:
THIS IS THE END; HOLD YOUR BREATH AND COUNT TO TEN 173

ACKNOWLEDGEMENTS:
THANK YOU FOR BEING A FRIEND 177

ABOUT THE AUTHOR:
IF THEY ASKED ME, I COULD WRITE A BOOK 180

INTRODUCTION

As humans, we tend to be on the lookout for shortcuts or quick fixes to our problems. Just one look at the diet and fitness industry proves that tendency. No one wants to lose weight the slow and steady way; we want a quicker solution, something that will bypass the discomfort of dieting and the ridiculous amount of endurance and willpower required to achieve our weight-loss goals.

The same is true for vocal health. Everyone who loses their voice goes on a mad dash to find the cure, the quick fix, the solution that will allow them to get back to life as usual because nobody has time to go on vocal rest.

Before I continue any further, this book is NOT about how to CURE voice loss and vocal fatigue. Rather, it's about preventing voice loss and vocal fatigue from ever happening at all. There are no quick fixes for vocal damage; once the voice has been damaged, vocal rest (or surgery) is the only way to heal the damage. This fact is the reason

I'm so hardcore about singers knowing how to prevent it in the first place.

Voice loss prevention has been a consistent passion project of mine for over 20 years, yet I still feel like I'm just scratching the surface of influencing the performance industry that a solution exists for voice loss and vocal fatigue. Until it is widely known and accepted that voice loss is preventable, until knowing how to prevent it is normalized, and until it's extremely rare for a major recording artist to let down fans by canceling a month of concerts because of voice loss, I'm likely to continue to feel as though I'm holding onto a big secret.

My goal is to be the go-to vocal health expert for recording artists who suffer in the studio, struggle on tour, and have close relationships with their ENTs who are armed with steroid shots, should these artists reach out in need. It breaks my heart when I hear about recording artists who struggle and consider major surgery on their precious vocal cords because they don't understand how to protect their voices. It makes me cry when I hear another recording artist canceled a series of shows due to voice loss even though I don't have a ticket to the show or know any of their music. I cry because I know how it feels to back out of a series of shows because I can't perform, and I wouldn't wish it on anyone.

I'm passionate about helping major recording artists in particular because they experience voice loss the most frequently, largely because of the demands of touring and studio recording schedules. When someone isn't armed with the tools I want to share with you, but they have a schedule that demands a lot from their voice, they are more susceptible to voice loss and vocal fatigue. However, armed with my Unlimited Vocal Health™ System, even the craziest schedule becomes irrelevant once voice loss is a non-issue.

If you think you are in the wrong place because you're not a big-time recording artist, I want to set you straight. This book is for you if:

- Vocal fatigue or voice loss prevents you from experiencing the life you desire
- You feel tired after using your voice for an extended period of time
- You feel tired after using your voice with more volume than is typical
- Voice loss is more normal to you than a healthy voice
- You have never experienced any signs of vocal fatigue or voice loss and you want to keep it that way

And of course, if you happen to personally know a big-time recording artist who struggles with vocal fatigue and who could benefit from this information, I would love you forever if you are willing to make an introduction.

So, rest assured, you've come to the right place, and you've learned why the topic of vocal health is so near and dear to my heart. After reading this book, you may find you want more custom help implementing what you've learned, and I'd love to coach you. The best place to start the coaching process is **www.getmypowerup.com**.

Another group I coach is fellow voice teachers or singers wanting to become voice teachers. I offer a training & certification program for teachers wishing to teach my vocal method to their own clients. If this is you, **www.getmypowerup.com** is also the best place for you to get started.

Keep an eye out for some free stuff as you move ahead in this book. I've put several free resources in here to supplement the reading. That way, you can feel as supported as possible. So, you will want to grab those tools when you see them.

You'll also see a place in each "part" which I call the "Bullshit Breakdown." It's a section where I list a lot of false information you may have heard about singing, speaking, and vocal health, which is complete bullshit. Then, I explain why it's bullshit rather than truth. What you read in this book may surprise you, and it may even trigger you. I encourage you to remain open-minded as that is the best way to learn new habits.

To prevent voice loss FOR GOOD, you'll learn my three-step system that must be mastered to achieve lasting results. Individually, each of these three steps is an excellent component of singing, but voice loss prevention will not be possible to achieve without a mastery of all three steps working together.

Another important note: the same three steps you master for your singing are required for your speaking voice too, or you'll still be susceptible to voice loss. But not to worry, there's a whole chapter devoted to learning how to prevent voice loss in your speaking as well.

Lastly, I'll share some of my favorite vocal health tips. Almost 100% of the time when I share this advice with clients, I am met with a litany of, "but what about XYZ...?" They question possible exceptions to what I present. So, prepare yourself to have that initial response. But keep in mind that once you get to that chapter, you'll have learned how to PERMANENTLY prevent voice loss. The questions that arise in you and the certain what-if scenarios you'll conjure up in your mind come from the place of fear you likely felt before opening this book – back when you believed voice loss was something you were doomed to endure if it decided to appear on your doorstep.

So, when those thoughts and fears arise, I invite you to take a nice, relaxing, low breath and remind yourself that all these vocal health tips are just a bonus I give you rather than a how-to guide for surviving your next bout of voice loss. That's because once you implement what you've read in this book, voice loss will no longer be a struggle for you. You'll have uncovered THE SECRET.

PART I

FOUNDATION

VOCAL CORE POWER

CHAPTER ONE

EVERY BREATH YOU TAKE

"Sometimes the most important thing in a whole day is the rest we take between two deep breaths."

– Etty Hillesum

When I was a sophomore in high school, I'd been in choir and private voice lessons a little over a year. My voice teacher, Mrs. Mueller always emphasized the importance of being aware of what was going on in my belly when I sang. I really did TRY to understand what she told me, but I was too eager to sing, so her instructions went in one ear and out the other.

But on that particular day, I had an epiphany in my bathroom before school. As I bent down to turn on the faucet in my tub to start my shower, I suddenly felt my little pooch of a belly cave to the magical powers of gravity. I felt it drop into relaxation completely naturally. It was one of those cartoon moments where I'm certain a little animated lightbulb appeared on top of my head. "THAT'S what she meant!!", my brain reasoned, attempting to decipher Mrs. Mueller's mystic code from the previous year. She often told me to relax my belly, but as a teenager (hell, as a FEMALE!), that wasn't exactly something I felt eager to attempt. I spent the bulk of my life holding in my belly because I was socially brainwashed to believe a little pooch in the belly was unattractive and needed to disappear. Because this particular instruction required me to do something unattractive, I was pretty quick to dismiss it until I felt it relax on its own.

Growing up, I heard parents of people my age saying they hoped their kids would have children of their own who behaved just like they did as some sort of punishment. I didn't have kids, but I did become a voice teacher and found myself with plenty of "kids" just like me who preferred to dismiss instruction they didn't really like for one reason or another. Relaxing the belly was one of these particularly ignored instructions.

Let's connect the dots and be aware of what a relaxed belly has to do with your voice. In the very least creepy-stalker way possible, if you get the chance to watch a baby or toddler sleep, take a moment to pay attention to her breath. Noticing breathing patterns works on sleeping adults too. It's just somehow easier to see (and get away with watching) on a small child. Once the child is asleep, you'll see the belly button region going out and in with the breath. The belly goes out as air is taken in, filling the space inside, and the belly goes in as the air is expelled, emptying the space inside. While this movement may not sound like a revolutionary concept, if you ask that same kid when awake to show you what it looks like to take the biggest breath possible, something very different will happen. The chest of the child will puff up, and possibly even the shoulders will raise up to the ears, arms frequently raised in the air as well. Once the child goes back to sleep, that breath will go back to happening in the belly again.

Odd, right? Our conscious understanding of what happens when we breathe is the direct opposite of what actually happens when we breathe without being conscious of breath. Whether we are so accustomed to holding in our bellies all day long that relaxing them seems unnatural, or whether we have adopted a vague understanding that breath happens in the lungs which live in the chest, the way we breathe when we think about how it's done drastically varies from the way we breathe when we aren't thinking about how it's done.

When we relax the belly muscles and let them hang out just like they did when I turned on the tub faucet that morning, we allow our rib cage – which is what houses our lungs – more room to expand so that a big breath is possible. However, if we inhale without first relaxing the belly, in addition to creating unnecessary tension, we limit the capacity of the lungs to inhale as much air as is required to sing an entire phrase. The breath has nowhere to go which is why it fills up in the chest.

Just like relaxing the belly creates more space for your lungs to expand, tightening the belly takes away potential space for your lungs to expand. And that's not all. When you inhale with a tightened belly, you require more breaths – which are smaller breaths – to make up for the inability to take the big breath you need. Taking too many small, shallow breaths can cause the body to believe it's in trauma or panic-mode. I'm sure you'd agree it's pretty challenging to have an effective performance if your body feels panicked.

In case it's not obvious, you need a bigger breath in singing than you do in speaking because the words you sing are elongated. When spoken, the same text as the lyric of a song will take considerably less time to get all the way to the end. It's why you rarely have to think about when you're going to take a breath when speaking. You can pretty much guarantee your body will instinctively take enough of an inhale. However, when singing, we need to make sure we have plenty of air to complete the lyric. So, our bodies enough space inside to take in a than we normally do just for

This type of breath is called a "low breath" in the singing industry. The type that happens in the chest because of a tightened belly is referred to as a "shallow breath."

With all that information in mind, the first step to taking a breath large enough to allow for a lengthy phrase is to relax the belly. Try not to get frustrated if this concept doesn't really make any sense to you right now. I will show you some helpful tips so your breath can take up more space than you're accustomed to currently.

One of the easiest ways to relax your belly so that you can take a bigger breath is to lie on your back. The reason it's easier this way is, much like the tub situation I had, gravity takes over and allows your social instinct that wants to tighten to have a little break. Find a spot on the floor to lie on your back, then bend your knees with your feet flat on the floor. Or you can even do this exercise on your back in bed. Put a hand on your chest and another hand on your belly, close your eyes, and just observe what happens.

In the beginning, you may still breathe in the shallow regions, but once your body relaxes more, you'll notice that your breath naturally happens in the low region where we want it to happen. I often say that singing requires undoing bad habits so we can get back to what our bodies were designed to do naturally: just BE. This breathing practice is a perfect example of our bodies doing what they were intended to do on their own. Instinct is why the child breathes correctly when sleeping (and why you do, too); it's the natural way to breathe. The trick is getting your body to breathe this way when you're standing up which requires more – you guessed it – relaxation.

But before you get back up, let's make sure you can breathe with a relaxed belly when you take in a big breath on purpose. Until now, we've only observed what our breath does when left to its own devices, so let's see if we can keep it grounded in nature when we ask it to do something specific.

Lie still on your back with a hand on your belly and a hand on your chest. Try to take in a larger breath than you normally would and see if it still comes in low or if you resort back to a chesty, shallow breath. Your air will come up into the chest toward the very end of the breath, we just don't want it to fill the chest region until the very end.

Once you've got that method down, try to take in a big breath – still on the floor – and then exhale it saying, "shh," like you're telling someone to be quiet. Sustain the "shh" until you completely run out of air. Then relax, take another deep and low breath, and "shh" it out till there's nothing left.

Speaking of nothing left, I'll share a cool trick you can try to further observe your body's instinct to breathe correctly. Read through the instructions first, and then go back to try it.

With a hand on your belly and a hand on your chest so you can feel where you inhale, exhale all the air you currently have in your body. Keep exhaling, even if you think you got all your breath out. Keep exhaling until the point you are concerned you might turn purple, and then allow yourself to inhale. That inhale will feel like a desperate gasp for air because you deprived your body from inhaling for so long. In its most desperate state, in order to take in the most air possible and rectify the situation of having no air at all, your body will breathe correctly. ALL that air will come rushing into the lower region of your torso. Cool, huh?

Ready to try this practice standing up?

I know it feels discouraging after having some success with this exercise to learn that your body tends to go back to its old tricks once you stand up. But here's the good news: in just this short amount of time, you've already developed some body awareness which is crucial to preventing voice loss for good. This newly found body awareness will keep you on track moving forward.

Speaking of body awareness, keep your hand-on-belly, hand-on-chest posturing until breathing low becomes second nature for you. You may also choose to close your eyes to deepen your awareness of your body's movements. In the standing position, observe your breath just like you did on your back. Take note of whether your body is breathing correctly now that you're standing or if it went back to shallow breathing. If you went back to the old habit, spend more time relaxing with eyes closed, observing your breath until you are relaxed enough for the breath to come in low like you want. And try to be patient – it WILL come.

Many components of singing require building muscle memory. If you've sung a long time and did so with bad habits, you first must break those bad habits so you can replace them with ideal habits. Your body may have to completely rewire its muscle memory. Just like when someone makes the switch to a Mac from a PC, they have to learn how to close a window on the left side of the screen after a lifetime of closing it on the right side (I dare you to pry my PC out of my cold, dead hands). In order to train their muscle memory, I assign my clients exercises to do between sessions. I DO NOT consider them "warm-ups" because each exercise has a specific purpose which is designed to – with repetition – aid in the rewiring of your body's muscle memory. You probably learned to ride a bike as a kid, and when you first learned, you had to keep practicing it so you wouldn't fall. But no matter how old you are or how long it's been since you've been on a bike, your body just knows how to ride it like you never took a break. The same is true with singing: you have to keep practicing your technique so your body will learn how to do it more instinctively.

I recommend doing the "Shh exercise" multiple times per day. This practice will allow you to increase your body's awareness of where the breath comes in, how to take large breaths correctly, and how to feel the sensation of using every bit of your air.

Another simple exercise I recommend is that every night while you're in bed, but before you fall asleep, put a hand on your chest and a hand on your belly and pay attention to what area moves and what doesn't. Really feel the sensation in your body and under your hands. Try to take a deep breath and keep it low. Do this process again before you get out of bed in the mornings.

Using these exercises will allow you to feel what's natural and to try and incorporate it into your daily life. Whenever possible, try to be sure you breathe low before speaking or singing. Make it your priority to master low breathing.

CHAPTER TWO

SING OUT LOUD, SING OUT STRONG

"Good physical condition is protection.
Our strength comes from our body."

– Jane Fonda

Because there's such an array of misinformation out there, it's always entertaining to discover what singers know and don't know about the topic of supporting the sound before working with me. One winter, I lived in New Jersey but commuted once a week to NYC and offered workshops to singers and actors. When I offered my class on supporting the sound, my entertainment factor was taken to a new level.

I have this philosophy that if a singer doesn't understand an element of technique clearly enough to explain to me how to do it, then they don't understand the element of technique clearly enough to perform it themselves when they're on their own. If they don't understand it well enough to do it when I'm not with them, it's highly unlikely that they'll use the technique at all.

"Tell me what you know about support, or what you think of when I use the phrase 'supporting the sound,'" I asked my NYC class that winter, just like I always begin when teaching on the topic of support. In my more than 20 years of experience teaching vocal technique, I've not once had a singer give me the correct answer. I like to ask this question in order to gauge their level of understanding on the topic of support. Plus, the answers I get entertain me. Inevitably, someone will blurt out incompletely, "Your diaphragm?" I've learned "diaphragm" is the go-to reply for questions singers don't know how to answer. Somewhere in their training they learned the diaphragm existed, but they obviously didn't understand it. So, if they don't know the answer to a question I ask, they assume the answer must be "diaphragm." Notice that there's no information about the diaphragm offered or any explanation about what they mean by their answer, they just simply say, "diaphragm," which I find fascinating and very telling.

How many voice teachers out there teach about the diaphragm? What are they teaching about it, and why doesn't anybody seem to understand or remember any of it? Their singers are clearly not applying any of their instruction to their singing because they have no idea what the diaphragm is or does, so they can't utilize what they learned about it in their singing.

After the obligatory "diaphragm" response, I will sometimes get another favorite answer, "breath support." I'll just say that A) this is another term that no one seems to be able to explain to me when I ask for clarification, and B) breath and support are NOT the same thing. They are two separate elements of technique.

Okay, I will climb down from my soapbox, for now. I will provide more information about this nonsense in the Part I Bullshit Breakdown.

One particular workshop in NYC provided my favorite response to the question about support.

"I was always taught to just... squeeze... you know, 'down there'... like doing Kegels... when I sing. Is that what you mean?" I think my jaw hit the grand piano I leaned against. How could I respond to this answer? I've also heard that support means to squeeze your butt, use a good sound system, or various methods of using the breath.

I GET IT. The idea of support can be confusing. And we coaches all give totally different advice about supporting the sound, if anything at all. But even more importantly, because of the unmistakable lack of understanding among singers, I question whether vocal coaches fully understand the concept of support themselves. I think if vocal coaches understood, they'd be able to explain support in a way their clients would understand, retain, and implement into their singing. AND they'd be able to identify and correct their clients when they use the technique incorrectly. These vocal coaches seem to understand that support is important and that they should talk about it at some point, so they say a little blurb about it and then go on to teach other things. Their singers are lost and skip over one of the most crucial components of preventing vocal damage.

So, what is the correct answer? Supporting the sound allows the core abdominal muscles to take the initial impact of sound production so that the vocal cords can perform their only job: flapping together to make sound. Support is one of the most fundamental elements of singing and speaking. Period. A properly utilized support system gives four primary benefits which I call, "The Four Ps."

P #1 is PROTECT: This point is near and dear to my heart and deserves its position as the first P in the Four Ps. All four are important, but I've placed them in this order based on their contribution to a healthy voice.

One of the most important functions of your support system is its ability to protect your vocal cords from damage. Your vocal cords are tiny but mighty. Their sole purpose is to make sound by flapping together quickly.

When sound is made without engaging the support system, those tiny but mighty vocal cords take the brunt of the initial impact of sound production. They slam together at first before quickly flapping as intended. When you allow your support system to take the brunt of the initial impact of sound using the much larger and tougher muscles of your core, then the only job the cords have is to quickly flap together to make sound, which is exactly what they're meant to do.

Repeated slamming together by allowing the impact to be made at the vocal cords, however, causes your cords to swell and develop callus-like spots which prevent the cords from closing together properly. When the cords can't come together all the way, sound cannot be properly produced, which is what causes the singer or speaker to lose her voice.

P #2 is PROLONG: In the last chapter, I mentioned how in singing all the phrases are elongated and take much more time to complete. Because of that lengthening, we have to make sure we take a big breath, so there is enough air for the entire phrase. Once you learn how to utilize your support system, you might think this P seems counterintuitive because it will seem like you are forcing all your air out in one motion before you finish the first lyric of your phrase, but utilizing your support system helps you to regulate the air you take in, so you don't lose it too quickly. It helps the breath you take last longer.

P #3 is POWER: Remember when you were little, and you sat at the top of the stairs and scooted down each stair on your butt while making a sound like "ahhhh"? Every time you landed on another step, your voice would sort of jolt forward from the impact of hitting the stair, like "AAaaahhh, AAaaahhh, AAaaahhh". The bump was like a little boost of power to your voice, and it was HILARIOUS, which is why you kept doing it. You didn't force that added volume to your sound, hitting the stair is what caused it to happen.

Similarly, when you utilize your support system in your singing, your voice gets a little jolt of power, too, allowing your voice to have some extra power and volume without having to strain from your throat.

P #4 is PITCH CONTROL: This point is exclusively for singers. Utilizing your support system gives you added control when it comes to maintaining the center of the pitch. This means that if you tend to sing a little sharp or a little flat, your support system will give you grounding and more ability to control being in the center of the pitch.

Any of The Four Ps can lead to some serious problems with your voice if the support system isn't used. And, in my experience, most people don't utilize their support system. It's not that they're being rebellious or dismissive, it's because most people don't even know they have a support system, much less how to use it.

Have you ever laughed so hard that your abdominal muscles hurt like you just did a hundred crunches? That sensation is your body engaging your support system to protect you from losing your voice from laughing. Remember that taking a low breath is the way we naturally and organically breathe without consciously thinking about it. Our bodies take the driver's seat at certain times, like when we laugh, and engage the support system on our behalf so that we don't cause damage to ourselves. Another time it steps in on our behalf is when we cough or sneeze. Utilizing your support system for singing and speaking will most likely feel unnatural and odd at first, but it is a totally natural tool we can access on our own, outside of when our body innately deems it necessary.

Think about the kind of sound you would make if I were to punch you in the belly. I'm not the punching type, and it is impossible to execute a punch through this book, so you'll have to use your imagination. But a hard jab to your gut would sound something like, "huugh!"

Now, I want you to imagine how your posture would change if I told you that in a few moments a swimsuit photographer would walk in to take pictures of you in a bikini or a speedo. Did you immediately tuck in your belly to try and make it disappear?

Next, we're going to put those two actions together: tuck in your belly as if to make yourself look slimmer while making a sound like you're being punched in the belly. Something to watch during this exercise: make sure you don't add any extra raspiness or strain to your punch sound. The sound should be mostly tone/voice and nothing extra. If your throat feels scratchy when you make the sound, you're adding something unnecessary.

Let's try two of those sounds in a row. You're going to say, "Huh" twice while tucking in your tummy quickly and firmly as you say each one, and you'll relax your belly in between the two tucks. For the purposes of this exercise, don't take a new breath between the two tucks, just relax your belly.

The reason we relax the belly between the tucks is so we can get in the habit of relaxing to take a low breath. In the last chapter, we talked about the importance of relaxation when it comes to taking a low breath. Even though we won't take a breath between every tuck in our exercises, we WILL practice relaxing. I want you to practice relaxing your belly when you're not making sound, so it becomes second nature to you to do it – especially if you are someone like I was, and you tend stay tucked all day. Think of your belly being in the tucked position every time you make sound and being in the relaxed position every time you take a breath. In the instance of vocal exercises, relax every time you stop making sound, whether or not you take a breath.

Imagine we go into the bathroom, and I pick up a tube of toothpaste, unscrew the cap, and put the toothpaste tube on the counter. What would happen? This is not a trick question. The correct answer is that nothing would happen. Now imagine that after putting the tube of toothpaste on the counter, I made a big fist and pound my fist onto the tube without its cap. What would happen this time? You'd probably feel pretty irritated with me because the toothpaste would come squirting out, making a giant mess all over the bathroom!

In this scenario, think of your torso as a tube of toothpaste, my fist as your support system, and the toothpaste inside as your voice. I want you to imagine – just like the toothpaste sitting on the counter doing nothing – that if your support system isn't engaged, you cannot make sound even though we know it IS possible. With the support system engaged, like the pounding fist to the tube of toothpaste, your voice comes out strongly but effortlessly. This effortless sound happens because you allowed a bigger muscle group to take the impact of making sound rather than asking the little vocal cords (or the toothpaste) to do it themselves. In its simplest form, this illustration is what it looks like to support your sound.

Again, remember that when you make sound, you are in the tucked position. When you take a breath, you are in the relaxed position. This process applies 100% of the time that you use your voice, whether singing or speaking. This concept needs to be fully understood and implemented so that it can be committed to your muscle memory.

We left off in our practicing with doing two tucks with a relax in between, so let's keep going, resuming with three tucks, then four tucks, and then finishing with five tucks. I recommend doing these tucking exercises incrementally, adding another tuck each time you complete the previous set successfully, and it shouldn't take more than a minute or two to perform all the exercises.

Please be kind to yourself, especially if this exercise feels challenging. It requires a little bit of coordination, but once you get the hang of it, the method will become much easier. Remember that your tucks are tucks inward; they are NOT pushes outward. If your belly is pushing out, that's not correct. You want to tuck your belly inward. It's a lot like what a personal trainer might ask you to do while lifting weights or doing sit-ups.

Speaking of personal trainers, the few I've had have all been shocked by the number of crunches I'm able to do without difficulty. Looking at me, it's not obvious that I have a strong core, but because of all this work we do in singing, I do. I like to joke with trainers that I have a well-defined six-pack, but I keep mine insulated.

Once you get the hang of a low breath and how to support your sound, it's time to apply these elements to a song or to a piece of text. To illustrate this concept, if you sing "Mary Had a Little Lamb," for example, there's no need to tuck on each syllable of the song. Instead, relax and take in a low breath at the beginning of the line, then tuck as you sing "Ma-ry had..." and maintain that tucked belly all the way through the phrase until it's time to breathe again. Then, relax your belly, inhale, then tuck your belly as you continue, "Lit-tle lamb...," etc.

Breath and support are NOT the same thing, but they do work together. Both components are required to make consistent healthy sounds.

**My No Limits Academy clients have access to my entire anthology of training videos and there are several on the topics of breath and support. If you'd like to check them out, you can get a seven-day free trial of my Academy by visiting:

https://singwithoutlimits.com/membership/no-limits-academy-trial-membership/

CHAPTER 3

COME TOGETHER RIGHT NOW OVER ME

"Coming together is a beginning. Keeping together is progress. Working together is success."

– Henry Ford

When I started dating after my husband of 17 years left me (Read about it in my 1st bestselling book here: **www.turnsoutimhot.com**), meeting someone with whom I had a strong connection was very important to me. But what does that connection mean, exactly? For me, it meant that the essential pieces of my personality needed to complement the essential pieces of his personality. I wanted us to feel like we belonged together. True connection meant that, even though we were incredible, whole, and badass individually, we were even stronger together.

People become couples all the time without this kind of bond. I'm pretty certain my ex and I never had a connection like that. So, it's not like a relationship CAN'T happen without one, it's more like everything is just a million times better when that connection is there.

Just like a relationship CAN happen without the beautiful connection, singing and speaking can happen without the sound being connected to the breath. When this happens, the person making sound holds her breath and makes sound at the same time. This issue not ideal, and it can be very frustrating for the singer who usually has no idea of her problem. Yet holding your breath while singing is possible, and it happens far more often than you might think. In fact, you may do it yourself and not even be aware of it. When a singer holds her breath while singing, it means that her breath – even if it's a low breath – and her tone are not connected. It also frequently means that her support system is not being utilized.

This lack of connection is a form of unwanted tension in the body that becomes habitual for the singer or speaker who makes sound while holding her breath. Singing or speaking while holding your breath can cause all kinds of other tension too. It typically ends up leading to a tendency for shallow breathing because a trauma situation is created in the body. The singer will almost always feel as though she's running out of breath, even though she has so much air left after completing a phrase.

If you find that you always feel short of breath when you sing or speak, or if you find that you expel a bunch of air after you sing or speak, these are the two most common signs that you are holding your breath while you make sound. When this occurs, your breath and your tone are not connected, and typically, your breath and support systems are not working together properly.

Especially since this information is probably all new to you, it's understandable if all the elements don't work together properly just yet. To avoid creating bad habits moving forward, there's an easy way to check if you are holding your breath when you sing or if you are breathing and supporting your sound correctly. This exercise helps determine if your sound and your breath are connected.

If you are unable to flutter your lips (think "motorboat") while making sound, it is a good sign that you are holding your breath. It also means that your breath and support aren't yet totally coordinated, or "connected."

If you are punched in the belly, the resulting sound typically starts with "H" because your breath is forced out. When I work with my private clients, I frequently ask them to start certain words or phrases with the letter "H" if I sense that they are not fully connecting their sound to their breath. Producing an "H" sound requires breath, so to do your tucking support work on syllables that start with an "H" allows your body to start the habit of making a connection between your breath and your support immediately.

When working on a song, I suggest that my clients sing the entire song on a vowel sound (like "ay") beginning with an "H" (like "Hay"). This practice develops the habit of connecting their breath to their tone from the beginning of the song-learning process. Then, once they start singing using the actual text of the song, it's much easier to keep that connection going, even on words that don't begin with an "H" because they created a habit.

These three pieces of technique: low breath, support, and connection comprise the Vocal Foundation, and they make up the first step of preventing voice loss.

Work on these three elements of foundation diligently until they become part of your muscle memory, until it's harder to sing incorrectly than it is to sing correctly. Make sure you don't just work on the exercises; always apply what you do in the exercises to actual songs, or you'll become someone who is FABULOUS at executing vocal exercises, but who struggles with application to a song.

While breath, support, and connection all need to exist in your vocal technique to have a solid foundation, know that foundation alone isn't enough to permanently prevent voice loss. The foundation is merely the first step in a process that requires ALL the steps to work.

If you'd like some additional support to make sure you're on the right track, I'd love to invite you to check out No Limits Academy using a free trial membership. You can grab yours at:

www.singwithoutlimits.com/coaching/no-limits-vocal-academy/.

PART I

THE BULLSHIT BREAKDOWN

There's A LOT of bullshit out there when it comes to singing and to vocal health. I created the Bullshit Breakdown because you may decide to take what you learn in this book and ask another coach about it or find out what your choir director has to say. It's very likely that you will encounter a lot of opposing thoughts about what is written in these pages. I have experienced this conflict my entire career. But what I know to be true is that for more than two decades, the components of my vocal method, Unlimited Vocal Health™, have created hundreds of singers that not only NEVER lose their voices, but allow them to perform in ways that other singers think must be superhuman.

The people who oppose my methods do not have the same results.

I often am asked to provide "translations" for my clients when they are given critiques or direction from heads of projects they are involved with. It's fairly common, albeit unfortunate, for singing competition judges, theatrical music directors, and even prior vocal coaches or choir directors to lack accurate information or training on the voice. So, when these judges are required to give feedback to one of my singers, my client and I often have to sit down with the critique and figure out what the critic intended, since they used terminology that doesn't make logical sense in their feedback.

For example, thanks to Randy Jackson on *American Idol*, competition judges will often say that a singer is "pitchy" when they are, in fact, singing accurately in tune. Typically, this judge noticed that something was off about the performance, but they couldn't place what it was, so they instead threw out the *Idol*-bred term, "pitchy." We then review the performance, when possible, and see if we can identify what they might have thought was off about that performance.

Similarly, an actor might come to me with feedback from their music director who asked them to sing a certain portion of their song "in a chest voice." This request (as you'll learn in PART II) makes no sense at all in contemporary music. So, let me translate for you here of some of the bullshit you may have heard in your experience.

Let's break down the BULLSHIT when it comes to Vocal Foundation, shall we?

THE DIAPHRAGM

This term is an evergreen, plentiful resource for bullshit. Allow me to be completely transparent and let you know that I used to talk about the diaphragm in the ways I mention below before I dug in a little deeper. I once had a teacher that told me it was my diaphragm that provided the support — two teachers, actually. When I looked into the source of support on my own years later, I discovered the truth and quickly made a correction.

WHAT THE DIAPHRAGM DOES

When you take a low breath, your diaphragm, a dome-shaped muscle that lives inside your rib cage at the base of your lungs, moves down to get out of the way so your lungs have more room to expand and take in air. When you exhale, it moves back up, helping to rid all the air from your lungs. The diaphragm creates a sort of vacuum seal that regulates the air going in and out of the lungs.

THE END.

Your diaphragm performs this function whether you want it to or not. You cannot control it, even if someone tells you to try.

WHAT THE DIAPHRAGM IS NOT, DOES NOT, AND CANNOT DO

ANY of the BULLSHIT listed below is what you will hear people say, ad nauseum:

- Breathe from your diaphragm
- Breathe into your diaphragm

- Breathe through your diaphragm
- Strengthen your diaphragm
- Push from your diaphragm
- Speak from your diaphragm
- Use your diaphragm
- Sing from your diaphragm
- Engage your diaphragm
- Sing through your diaphragm
- Project from your diaphragm

And my personal favorite came from a judge who we "think" complimented my client when he told her he "observed a tighter diaphragm."

When you hear someone saying something like these pieces of pure bullshit, and you're not yet one of my clients, my best advice is for you to ask that person, as sincerely as possible, if they can demonstrate or explain what their request means. Then brace yourself for whatever might come after that.

Remember, if someone isn't able to explain how they execute a certain element of technique, they probably don't fully understand how they do it themselves. Teachers, judges, and directors will often use terminology they don't fully grasp, so if you ask them to demonstrate what they advise, it's not often they'll be able to demonstrate it. They may know enough to know that something seems off, they just may not know exactly what it is.

Besides the fact that this practice spreads bullshit like wildfire, the other reason I take issue with it is that in some cases, poor advice can hurt a singer. If the critic gives bullshit feedback, and the singer doesn't recognize it's bullshit, they may attempt to "correct" themselves and cause damage to their voice.

BREATH SUPPORT

I wish I could insert a "face palm" emoji at this point in the book. This "term" is complete BULLSHIT. What the diaphragm actually does is help your lungs to inhale and exhale more efficiently. Remember that breath and support ideally work together, but they are two very different, very specific functions. "Breath support," however, isn't a real thing. Your support system supports your sound/your voice/your cords; it does not support your breath, which doesn't need support. Your breath is prolonged when you utilize your support system, but your breath isn't supported by your support system. Here are some of the ways you will hear this made-up term used as a piece of attempted legitimate advice:

- Work on your breath support
- Maximize your breath support
- Use more breath support
- Breath support would fix your problem
- Control your breath support
- This lacks breath support

Recognize that when someone uses this bogus term that they likely don't fully understand what they are talking about and, like with the diaphragm, they will struggle to demonstrate or describe this term in detail. My best advice to you when you hear this term thrown around is to imagine the person saying, "unicorn," instead of, "breath support." Both ideas are made up, so it's practically the same thing, really.

Just kidding! My actual advice in this situation is to ask for clarification: ask if they are referring to your breathing OR to supporting your sound. Then, I'd ask for clarification on what specifically is wrong, incorrect, or lacking about it. I've found that a lot of times people using this term "breath support" are referring to just the breath. This is another reason I think support is so unknown; it is being lumped in as breath when support is actually its own separate function – one of the most important functions of making healthy sound.

If you would like some help making sense of all the bullshit, I'd love to chat with you about what it looks like to work with me.

You can schedule that chat using my application here: **www.getmypowerup.com**.

PART II

PLACEMENT

LIMITLESS POWER & RANGE

CHAPTER 5

TOO LEGIT TO QUIT

"We break a lot of rules. It's unheard of to combine opera with a rock theme, my dear."

– Freddie Mercury

I fell in love with singing around age four or five in the little front room of our house that had a stereo system and a record player. The three singers/bands I remember first were: Kenny Rogers, Queen, and Survivor. I knew several of Kenny Rogers' songs by heart and completely fell in love with him. I liked the warmth of his voice and thought he seemed like a teddy bear. I didn't have the best relationship with my dad and I remember wishing Kenny Rogers was my dad. I also loved Queen's "Another One Bites the Dust" and Survivor's "Eye of the Tiger." I loved the beat of both of these songs and my young, literal mind was mystified by the meanings of the lyrics.

The first time I experienced *classical* music was as a piano player. I got my piano when I was five years old. At the time, all the neighbor kids had pianos and took lessons. I've never been one to follow the crowd, but the first time I heard my neighbor's piano, I fell in love and wanted to take lessons immediately. I wasn't a particularly good piano player, but I enjoyed playing. I just wanted to learn piano so I could accompany myself, because all I REALLY wanted to do was SING.

Classical music was beautiful to me, but it was a totally different world than the kinds of songs I wanted to sing. When I got to high school, I sang classical music in choir and in my private voice lessons, and I developed an appreciation for it.

One thing I noticed back then - that I just figured would change with time - was that when I sang the songs I loved from the radio, I didn't sound like the people I heard on the radio. Instead, the sound I made was more like when I sang in choir or in my private lessons. There was a "stuffiness" about the choir music and my solo repertoire from my lessons that I didn't want to be there when I sang songs by Debbie Gibson, Heart, or Whitney Houston. I was observant enough to recognize that they were two totally different sounds, but I was only trained to create the classical type of sound.

I developed a very strong classical singing voice and won several scholarships as a result. My college private voice teacher really wanted me to go into opera, but I had my sights set on Broadway. We worked on a lot of classical music together with an occasional musical theatre piece thrown in. The musical theatre pieces she assigned me, however, didn't really step outside of operetta. They were quite formal, which left me feeling unsatisfied since I longed to be singing all my favorite Broadway hits, like "Adelaide's Lament" from *Guys & Dolls*, or "At the Ballet" from *A Chorus Line*.

When I went to my acting conservatory in NYC, I learned that classical singing is referred to as "legit" in the musical theatre world. There were two other techniques called "belt" and "mix" that

I'd never heard of before that would help me achieve the sound I longed to sing.

In musical theatre, "legit" music was reserved for the classics, the ingenue roles, the classier leading lady roles. These were the kinds of roles I'd longed to work on in college, but instead had to work on the only musical theatre pieces that were reminiscent of opera, like "Vilia" from *The Merry Widow*, and "Letter Song" from *Ballad of Baby Doe*. I later discovered that, technically, "legit" roles (including Julie Jordan from *Carousel*, Hodel from *Fiddler on the Roof*, or Marian from *The Music Man*) didn't even use a true classical technique, but rather a more formal version of the "mix" technique.

The other two techniques - belt and mix, which we'll cover in the next two chapters – sounded dramatically different than the classical sound I'd learned up to that point. While they didn't quite sound like the radio sound I aimed for in high school, they seemed a bit closer than the classical stuff I learned for years.

At first, I was extremely hesitant to learn belt & mix. Belt was very loud which made me concerned it must be dangerous. I sat in my vocal technique class with crossed arms and a visible scowl on my face, absolutely refusing to damage my voice in the ways my instructor was surely encouraging us to do. Stubbornly and completely devoid of trust, I decided I was only willing to work on legit technique because I wasn't interested in destroying my voice which I was convinced would happen. In retrospect, it seems I've always been concerned about protecting my voice.

I ended up caving to learn belt & mix, but they didn't come easy for me at all. I went home and sat at the piano in my apartment with all my notes, trying to make sense of what my instructor taught us about these two, seemingly dangerous techniques. The one clear difference I noticed between classical technique and belt & mix techniques was that belt & mix were the opposite of classical in just about every way.

With my clients, I still teach classical technique, but I now refer to it as the "basic" technique. I can already see, hear, and feel all your feathers ruffling because I'm referring to something quite difficult to do as "basic," but let me explain. Because I primarily work with contemporary singers who have no intention of ever singing classical music, I consider classical technique to be the first step of many. I use classical technique primarily as a ground zero or a base on which to build their contemporary singing. For a contemporary singer with no intention of ever singing classical music, the classical technique offers a concrete way to develop body awareness of what NOT to do in contemporary singing. For these reasons, I call classical the "basic technique."

Contemporary singing requires getting back to what your body was designed to do organically in order to make sound AND stay healthy. Classical singing (not unlike classical dance) demands that singers approach the voice in a way that is not at all organic, natural, or second nature. The classical sound isn't like speaking at all, nor is it like the voice that comes out by default from a singer with no vocal training. Similarly, ballet isn't at all like walking or like the default way our bodies move without any formal instruction. Classical singing and classical dancing are styles that requires the body to step out of its comfort zone and try something completely different.

Ready to try it out?

I'd like you to yawn the biggest, most spacious yawn you can yawn.

Are you yawning yet? I can say the word "yawn" a few more times if it'll help.

While you are yawning, notice the huge space that is created by stretching into that yawn. Do you feel the stretch in your mouth and throat that goes up and back as you yawn? Notice also if you hear a deeper sounding breath with a yawn space in the back. If you struggle to understand what I'm asking, think for a moment about impersonating Darth Vader by inhaling and then exhaling on a whispered "kaw." Do you feel that big, cavernous space back at the back of your mouth?

When you make that space, the soft palate, which is the squishy part of the roof of your mouth (not the hard palate which is where the peanut butter gets stuck), lifts and creates more space in the back of the throat while simultaneously blocking off the passageway into the nose. When the soft palate blocks of the passageway into the nose, it means no sound can escape there.

This knowledge is important because in the classical technique (and ONLY in the classical technique), you have a chest register and a head register with breaks in between. These classical terms are based on where the sound resonates in your body. With a raised soft palate (like a yawn), if you make a loud, booming sound in a low place in your range, you will be singing in your chest register, or chest voice. If you place your hand on your chest as you do this, you'll feel the sound vibrating in your chest.

If you then, with a raised soft palate, make a loudish, high-pitched sound like you would if you were cheering for your favorite team, like, "woo-hoo!!" you should feel that sound sort of spinning around in your head. That happens because the sound resonates in your sinus cavities, bouncing off your skull. The only place you can feel your skull on the outside is your teeth. So, place your thumb underneath your top front teeth and make that sound again. Do you feel the vibration in your teeth? This is your head register, or head voice.

Your raised soft palate blocks off the passageway into your nose, so let's do a simple exercise to test that. If you raise your soft palate and make that high sound like you are cheering at a sporting event or are imitating an owl's hoot, you are in your head voice. If you repeat that exact same action but you plug your nose, you should sound the same as when your nose was not plugged. That is because your raised soft palate blocks off the passageway into your nose.

If, however, you say in your regular voice, "Hello, my name is _____," then repeat the phrase while plugging your nose, you will notice a dramatic difference. In this example, because the soft palate is not raised, the sound comes out of the nasal passageway. Therefore, this exercise is a fantastic way to check if your soft palate is raised or neutral.

The reason it's important to know if your palate is raised or neutral is because it determines whether or not you are in a safe zone when singing. In classical singing, the soft palate must be raised, but in contemporary singing, using belt & mix, the soft palate MUST be in its neutral position. In classical singing, the raised soft palate, which blocks off the nasal passage, is what creates the chest voice, the head voice, and the breaks. In contemporary singing, the neutral soft palate is what causes the sound to resonate in the nasal passage, and what eliminates the chest voice, the head voice, and the breaks.

The position of your soft palate – raised for classical technique and neutral for belt & mix and speaking – determines the "placement" of your sound.

The chest voice is only meant to go so high (F# above middle C for men, A above middle C for women). When a singer stretches the chest beyond that limit, she puts herself at risk for vocal damage. This risk of vocal damage is the primary reason contemporary singers experience voice loss and vocal fatigue – from applying classical principles to contemporary music.

It's so tempting for singers who only know classical technique to stretch the chest voice higher than it's meant to go because in contemporary songs, no one is interested in switching to a head voice because it lacks the power and strength of the chest. The chest voice CAN be stretched; it's possible, but it's just very dangerous. For many contemporary singers, this understanding sparks a major "aha moment" because they realize why they experience voice loss and vocal fatigue: they are singing in a classical technique and stretching the chest voice higher than it's meant to go.

It's important to remember that the ONLY way to be in your chest voice or your head voice is to raise your soft palate like a yawn. This raised soft palate is also the only action that creates "breaks" or "passaggios" in your voice. Those breaks are where your voice shifts from your chest register into your head register, much like a bike shifting gears. So, because the chest voice is only able to safely go so high before it must shift into the head voice – which isn't automatic, you have to do it manually and intentionally – it is vital that a singer is aware of whether the soft palate is raised.

Let me say that another way: The raised soft palate (like a yawn) required for classical singing is what creates the ability to place your sound in a chest voice or a head voice or to have breaks in the voice. If a singer raises the soft palate and places the sound in her chest voice, she must be aware of how high she can safely sing before risking vocal damage by not switching into her head voice. Because this switch in placement has to be done manually, without having perfect pitch or an instrument at all times, knowing where the safe zone ends can be a challenging task.

You may wonder why classical singers singing classical music aren't stressed out about the potential risk of this placement shift. It's because with classical music, it is both appropriate and expected — especially with females — for the singer to sing in a head voice. With contemporary singers, like those we hear on the radio, singing in the head voice is frowned upon because it sounds like classical singing (because it IS!). The chest voice sounds stronger and more passionate, so the tendency is to use the chest voice when singing contemporary music. Since the notes of contemporary songs typically go higher than the break, singers stretch the chest voice past its limit, which causes the singer to experience vocal fatigue or voice loss.

I like to teach my singers the very basics of classical technique because I want them to be intimately familiar with what the classical placements (chest and head) feel like. This way, when they sing the contemporary techniques of belt & mix, they know when they place their sound incorrectly. Outside of knowing how to know if a singer's technique is correct, I don't really work with the classical technique much because I find it useful only for teaching body awareness which is crucial for proper placement of sound.

Since this chapter is fairly technical, let me break down the main takeaways for understanding the classical technique:

- If you intend to be a contemporary singer (singing anything other than classical or opera), the primary purpose of learning how to use the classical technique is to develop body awareness so it is easier to detect if you are singing the contemporary techniques safely and correctly.

- To make a classical sound, the soft palate must be lifted like a yawn so that it blocks off the passageway into the nose.

- Placement of sound refers to where you decide to have your sound resonate – raising the soft palate allows you to place the sound in your chest or in your head (classical singing), keeping the soft palate in its neutral position allows you to place the sound in your nose (belt & mix singing and speaking).

- The sound for a classical technique either resonates in the chest cavity or in the sinus cavity, depending on where you choose to place it.

- The chest voice is limited in how high it can ascend (F# above middle C for men, A above middle C for women).

- Contemporary singers and their listeners do not like the sound of the head voice which is why there exists a temptation for singers who haven't learned belt & mix to push the chest voice higher than it's able to go.

- When the chest voice is pushed higher than its limit, the singer is at risk for vocal damage.

- Contemporary singing should NEVER be done using the classical technique, which is the **only** technique that utilizes the chest voice, the head voice, and breaks.

CHAPTER 6

SING OUT, LOUISE!

"I started singing when I started talking."

– Mariah Carey

I was terrified. And I didn't get it. On my subway ride home from my NYC acting conservatory, I went over everything my technique teacher told us in class, writing down every instruction I remembered. I was hopeful that when I got home my roommates would be gone so I could sit at the piano and figure it out.

I was in luck.

At the piano, I looked over my notes. I was confused because what my teacher called "belting" sounded so much like singing in a chest voice. But he said we could belt at least an octave past where we could sing in a chest voice. I was convinced belting would hurt and that it would annihilate my voice because I knew how dangerous it was to sing in a chest voice higher than I was designed to. But he said we wouldn't use a chest voice when belting. This technique used our voices in a different way, so the breaks in the voice (caused by raising our soft palates) would go away completely when we belted. Hmm...

I wasn't alone in my bewilderment. NO ONE understood how to belt from that class; we were all confused. Another challenging part for me was that because my instructor was a man, I couldn't hear what belting ought to sound like with my voice. He gave us examples of singers to listen to so we would understand how it should sound, but most of his suggestions weren't even true belting.

I continued to read my notes and tinker on the piano as I mustered up the courage to try out belting a few tunes, hoping the neighbors wouldn't mind. It was pointless to hope they wouldn't hear me because I ALWAYS heard them. We had an opera singer, a cellist, and Chip Zien, one of my all-time favorite Broadway actors in my building.

Several hours later, I GOT IT. It was like a light switch was flipped on for me. Once I figured out the technique in my body, it just clicked, and I understood how to consistently make a belt.

Belting was definitely loud, and I surprised myself by how high I could do it. But the biggest shock to me was that it didn't hurt at all.

Eager to see if I could make it work in a song, I feverishly pulled out my music books that contained songs I'd always wanted to sing. One after another after another, I belted easily and sang songs with a sound I didn't know I could make. My favorite part was that belting seemed to naturally add this extra burst of emotion to my songs. I've always described belting as a technique that allows you to emotionally sing from your toes.

Several years into teaching voice, I discovered that I apparently teach belting the same way I figured it out on my own at the piano; I don't teach belting the way that it was taught to me. My client, Joanna, learned how to belt from me, then a couple years later, she went to my same acting conservatory in NYC. She had several of the same teachers I had ten years prior, including the vocal technique teacher who taught me belting. On Joanna's first day of learning how to belt from my instructor, she called me the second the class ended and said, "Katti, I have NO IDEA how you learned to belt from what he taught. It was nothing like what you taught me, and I was the only one in the class that knew how to belt. But that was because I learned it from YOU!" So, somewhere between what the instructor taught me and my own translation of it several hours later, I created my own understanding of how to belt. I've since spent decades successfully teaching this technique to other singers.

I usually preface a singer who is about to belt for the first time with these warnings:

- We're going to be very loud – it's just part of the deal
- You're likely going to feel a little silly because of what I'm going to ask you to do

- I'm more interested in you doing it RIGHT than I am in you doing it PRETTY. We'll make it pretty once you know that you know that you know you're doing it right.

So, consider yourself warned as we begin to learn how to belt.

First, I'd like you to imagine that you're an angry little three-year-old toddler about to throw a tantrum. I want you to scrunch up your nose like you're mad or like something smells really stinky. With your nose scrunched and in your best impersonation of an angry toddler, I'd like you to imagine that some other little kid just took your favorite toy and ran off with it, so you call out to them, "HEY!" with a considerable amount of volume, keeping that scrunched up nose and that angry toddler voice. I warned you that you might feel really silly because of what I ask you to do, but please trust the process. Your future singing thanks you!

I'm certain we can all agree that if someone swiped your purse and ran off with it, you would never call out, "Hey! That's mine!" to the thief in your stuffiest, open-space-in-the-back, as if you're attempting your best British accent while holding a teacup with your pinky finger lifted in the air. Instead, you'd put some "oomph" behind your voice. Your volume would increase to a yell, and there would be a meatiness to your sound. I like to call this your "calling voice."

Belting is singing in your calling voice. It's also completely natural. Think about an infant crying her lungs out. That wailing is powerful and strong and can go on for hours, yet the baby never suffers any vocal fatigue from doing it. That's because she is using her calling voice; she's belting. The infant cannot even speak the word "belt," yet she executes a flawless belt each time she gets upset and cries. That's how instinctive and natural belting is. Not only that, but if you watch the baby's belly as she screams out her cries, you'll notice she also supports her sound.

When we make our scrunched-up nose and our toddler voice to find our belt placement, which I call our "baby belt." It's like a beginner belt. We sound like very young humans, and we tap into the same skills babies use to scream for hours without consequences.

My singers almost always ask if they'll always have to scrunch up their noses when they belt. My answer is always "no," however, if you look at most singers while singing big high notes, you will often notice they make this same face. I made a small collection here: **https://singwithoutlimits.com/scrunchface/** if you'd like to see what I mean.

We make that face because it's really hard to sing in a chest voice (a booming sound with a raised soft palate) when we scrunch our noses and widen our mouth shape, which means it's really hard to belt INCORRECTLY. If you make this sort of "calling voice" sound, but with a raised soft palate, you will tire out very quickly, especially if you take that strength higher than the chest voice's limit. This type of error in singing is the most common way singers lose their voices.

So, we use the scrunched-up nose with a toddler's calling voice when learning to belt, so we can make CERTAIN we are belting rather than singing in a chest voice. As long as we are belting, we have the same power as that crying infant.

Once we are certain that we can belt correctly and consistently, we can then learn how to make the belting sound amazing. As I always tell my clients: when you are learning how to belt, doing it RIGHT is more important than doing it PRETTY.

Let's begin practicing your belting technique. You've just yelled, "HEY!" to that jerk of a kid who swiped your favorite toy. Let's do it again. Remember, you want to scrunch up your nose like a mad toddler, then imitate the young, angry voice of that toddler when you loudly call out "HEY!" to the kid, who by now has a pretty good head start with your favorite toy. I typically ask my clients to do this with the following added phrases which you're welcome to try at this point: "NO FAIR!" "THAT'S MINE!!" "NOOOO!!"

If at any point, your voice feels scratchy or sore from doing this exercise, STOP. Then, let's figure out why. Typically, discomfort means that you are making space in the back of your throat — that it's so normal for you to make that space you have to think about it to NOT make the space. Other times, it can mean that you are adding in unnecessary sounds to your voice - like grindy rattles - which will cause your voice to feel like sandpaper in no time. So, make sure you're not adding anything unnecessary or creating space in the back of your throat before continuing. The rule with belting is that if it hurts, you're doing something wrong.

Once you've gotten the hang of the belt placement and how to make a consistent sound that is healthy, it's time to try singing in your belt. I recommend singing "HEY" on a triad when you're starting out because it's not very complicated and allows you to make small, ascending and descending interval jumps while practicing this new technique.

The ONLY element I want you to focus on is making sure you place your sound in your nasal passageway, which means: 1) make sure you're not allowing space to open up in the back of your throat, and 2) make sure you're not doing what I call "cheating," which is when we freak out and then wimp out as the pitches get higher. Know also that most everyone cheats in the beginning because belting high is scary the first couple times.

"Cheating" is technically singing in the mix technique when you intended to sing in the belt technique, but you got scared and mixed instead, typically because the pitches got really high. So, to avoid cheating, keep these points in mind:

- With belting, especially in the beginning, you must sing louder as you get higher

- When belting high notes, you want to think about your mouth getting wider as you get higher. Once you've widened all the way, you can begin to drop your jaw, just DO NOT raise your soft palate in the back of your throat – keep that scrunched nose so it'll be too hard to make this mistake.

Keep practicing belting on a triad with the goal of remaining in a belt placement the entire time – which is your calling voice that's made with a neutral soft palate – especially as you get higher. Then, ease into belting a song! Start small – maybe just work on mastering the chorus at first. If you're anything like me, once you get the hang of this technique, it will just "click" for you, and you'll want to sing every song you never thought you could sing before. Do it but be smart about it. Make sure you're ready and know how to correct yourself if something seems wrong or starts to hurt.

If you want some help, let's have a chat and see which one of my programs would best support you in making healthy belting part of your singing. My singers typically learn to belt very quickly, and it doesn't take long once you've gotten the hang of it to polish it and master it in your singing. When you're ready to take the next step, set up a time for us to chat here: **www.getmypowerup.com**.

CHAPTER 7

WISH I COULD BE PART OF THAT WORLD

"Being both soft and strong is a combination very few have mastered."
— Yasmin Mogahed

I have a confession: I'm a pretty classic definition of a "crazy cat lady." I currently only have one cat, and the most I've ever had at one time is two, but I treat cats as people – my cats and yours. As long as I can remember, I've made voices for other cats, regardless of whether or not they were in my family. The craziest thing is when I have full-on conversations with them. CORRECTION: the craziest thing is when I report to another human, the "funniest thing the cat said the other day."

So now that we have that embarrassing detail out of the way, this explanation might make a little more sense. Once, as I attempted to describe the mix technique to a singer, I explained that it was kind of like the voice I use when I'm pretending my voice is the voice of my cats – it's kind of like a cutesy "baby voice."

Mix is typically the easiest technique to sing, yet the most challenging to define and describe. Most healthy singing involves getting back to what we do instinctively and really, mix is no exception to that rule. In fact, I often describe mix as the "default singing voice." It's the voice that we typically use when singing absentmindedly, when learning a song for the first time, when we sing "Happy Birthday," and so on. It's the voice we typically reach for by default. Once we officially learn how to mix, we do it intentionally, but for many singers, first learning the technique feels like learning something we've been doing forever without really thinking about it.

Mix is also the technique used by all our favorite Disney princesses. I'm sure you've instantly conjured in your mind one of many songs sung by Disney princesses. Let's take *The Little Mermaid*'s Ariel for example. Her voice isn't big and beefy like a belt, and it's not stuffy and proper like a classical sound. It has familiar vowel sounds just like speaking (and just like belting), and she's able to make it have a pop-like sound, without the power and punch of a belt or the rigidity of classical.

I want to be clear that if you've heard of the "mixed voice," please know that it is something very different from what I'm talking about. "Mixed voice" is a classical term that I find highly confusing and not at all the same thing as the mix technique.

My technical description for the mix technique is that it is taking your classical head voice and moving it into your belt resonance. Meaning, if you make a classical sound in your head voice by raising your soft palate, and then you move that sound from your classical head voice into your belt resonance by lowering your soft palate into its neutral position, you will have a mix. The difference between a belt and a mix is that belt is in your calling voice. Both techniques resonate in the nose (as does your speaking voice), but one (belt) requires more effort and volume.

My very simple and non-technical description for it is cheating. But mix is only cheating if you intend to be belting. Oftentimes "cheaters" are able to understand the mix technique a little easier because they found it by mistake – by chickening out on a high note they meant to be belting.

In musical theatre, mix is extremely common. One of the reasons it is so common is that the majority of singers who believe they sing classically actually sing using a mix. Remember, when we raise the soft palate, it blocks off the passageway into the nose. The second that soft palate opens up, even the teeniest space in the back, the singer begins to mix. And it's considered a mix from that point all the way till the palate lowers to its neutral position, which is where it lives all the time unless you are singing classically.

Let's do one of my favorite mix-finding exercises, "Back to Front." In this exercise, I want you to make a fairly high-pitched sound on "aww" with a raised soft palate and a dropped jaw, which means you'll be singing classically using your head voice. Plug your nose to make sure your palate is lifted all the way. Then, unplug your nose and slowly start to relax your soft palate from its yawn stretch back to its neutral position, and then start to widen your mouth and scrunch your nose. Sustain the pitch on "aww" through this entire motion. Try it!

Did you notice how the sound changed from a hollow, stuffy, and open sound into a lighter, brighter sound? That whole journey from the back of your throat once the soft palate lowers even just a smidge, all the way to the tip of your nose with a widened mouth and a fully neutral soft palate is the spectrum of your mix. So, since the spectrum of mix starts the moment the palate no longer blocks the nasal passage, singers often confuse it with their classical voice. It can be difficult for listeners to detect the difference in the way it sounds, which is why I always tell my singers to pay attention to how their singing feels. We can always replicate how something feels, but because we hear our own voices differently than others, we can't rely on how it sounds.

If you listen to Laura Osnes sing "If I Loved You" from *Carousel* and then you listen to Kelli O'Hara sing the same song, you will hear two different styles of mixing – Laura's is more contemporary, and Kelli's is closer to a classical while still being a mix. Then, look up Anna Moffo singing the song to hear it in a true classical technique. One tiny move of the soft palate makes it classical. For this reason, singers in musical theatre often think they are singing in the classical technique when they're actually mixing at the far end of the spectrum.

I'm guilty myself. When my mom remarried, she asked me to sing at her wedding, but because I'd been teaching singers daily how to belt and mix, I found myself singing her two chosen classical pieces in a mix by mistake. My muscle memory was very used to making a mix shape rather than a full classical shape, so I had to retrain my muscle memory and be sure to pay extra attention to what I was doing in order to use my classical technique for these songs.

This reason is why I prefer to teach mix last of the three techniques. Belt is SO different than classical that it's an easier comparison to classical – it's easier to know when belt is correct vs. incorrect because belt and classical are nothing alike. Mix has aspects in common with belt and elements in common with classical, so it can be much more confusing to learn mix without the benefit of first understanding belt. I've also found that learning mix first can make a singer who prefers to stay in the comfort of their mix a very timid belter.

Not only does mix have a huge spectrum of sounds it can create, but it also has a wide variety of uses in singing. The more classical-sounding version of mix is used in musical theatre as if it is classical, likely because it is a value of musical theatre as a whole to be familiar and understood. Classical vowel shapes make diction a bit tricky but softening into a mix even just a bit makes the vowels much closer to spoken tones which are easier to understand. There's also a much brighter, more forward version of mix that is used everywhere else in musical theatre where the singer isn't belting.

In the contemporary singing world, mix is used in the softer, more vulnerable parts of pop and R&B songs, as well as on the occasional high note in these genres. It's also frequently used in jazz, and it's occasionally used in folk and rock. The only country singer I've ever heard use a mix is Alison Krauss who is technically a bluegrass singer. Otherwise, country singers are typically belters. Belt is used in just about every genre.

I have a theory that one of the main reasons it's so common to hear the mix technique in pop music is that untrained singers who don't know how to navigate high notes switch into what they thought was a classical head voice when the pitches got high, but it was actually a mix. The way to know the difference between your classical head voice and your mix is recognizing whether your soft palate is raised or in its neutral position. This awareness is why developing body awareness is so crucial to healthy singing.

The practice of navigating high notes by switching into something easier, softer, and lighter (which was a mix) is a stylized choice singers make on purpose. If you've heard a pop singer who sounds like she's totally feeling her song in a powerful way and then, suddenly switches into a lighter, airy sound, that's often a conscious decision. I believe mix is a default decision among untrained singers who don't know how to stay strong. In other words, they don't know how to belt.

Curiously, when a singer uses a mix because she doesn't know how to remain strong, it's usually frowned upon as being a wimpy or ugly choice. Yet somehow, using a mix in this way turned into a trend and singers do all the time. So now, I teach singers how to make this conscious decision to pull back on a high note that they're fully capable of belting as a simple style choice. I tell them we don't want their voice to sound like they "can't" belt it, we want it to sound like they "chose not to" belt it.

My uncle designs illusions for famous magicians, which has always been pretty cool to me. He taught me what sleight of hand was when I was young. In the world of magic and illusions, a magician is able to deceive the audience into believing something happened magically because of some tricky, deliberate, and often quick hand movements that were well-rehearsed in advance. The result is that the audience members think "magic" is the only explanation for what happened seemingly right before their eyes.

Sleight of hand is something we can use in singing as well! I created a cool use for mix which I refer to as a "vocal sleight of hand" called "Mix Like Belt." Another handy trick of mix is its ability to make your audience think you are belting extremely high notes – which makes them wildly impressed by your skills – when you're actually just mixing, something that requires almost no effort on your part. The reason mixing is a handy part of the vocal health puzzle is that oftentimes if a note is too high for a belt to sound pretty – and I'm talking stratosphere-kind-of-high-belting – a singer may attempt to continue belting until the notes sound pretty-ish.

High belt notes require a lot of space and volume. When a belt note requires so much space and volume that it ceases to sound pretty, I typically decide instead to mix the note using the Mix Like Belt version I invented because it tricks your audience.

Let's explore Mix Like Belt. Think of a really high pitch in your head. Now, imagine that you are going to belt this pitch – don't do it, just imagine it. What all would be required of you and your body in order to belt this pitch? You would take a more solid stance and a much bigger breath. Your mouth would be open in every possible direction. Your nose would be scrunched, and you would be extremely loud.

Now, let's imagine that you are just mixing the same pitch – what is required of you and of your body this time? You wouldn't require any special stance. You could mix it while taking a nap or twisted up like a pretzel during a yoga class. Mixing it wouldn't require any more air than usual, nor would it require opening your mouth very much or scrunching up your nose. It definitely wouldn't require extra volume. In fact, you could likely mix this pitch perfectly in one quick sound that almost no one would be able to hear. This difference is because your belt is your calling voice, and your mix doesn't require the same amount of effort.

BUT... if I were in a big, powerful, belty moment in a song and the top note felt a smidge too high to belt while still sounding like I'm singing, causing me to sound a bit more like a squealing pig or an angry toddler, and I chose to mix the pitch instead, I would sound as though I asked my stunt double to come in and sing the pitch for me because the mix would sound NOTHING like the previous belt notes. This mix lacks the power, volume, and space that the belt requires. The mix sounds polished and easy whereas the belt notes sound powerful and difficult. Also, it is very anticlimactic to "wimp out" (cheat) on the top note in a powerful moment. So, this is when I would implement "mix-like-belt."

The way to do it is to physically go through all the motions we described that we'd make if we were belting it, but we would mix it instead. Meaning, we would mix the pitch with a huge mouth, a scrunched nose, and tons of volume, but we would NOT sing it in our calling voice. This little bit of "sleight of hand" in your singing will cause your audience to believe you belted the note. To be clearer, they may not think, "Wow! She belted that big top note!" Instead, they WON'T think, "OH! Hmm...that sounded... different..." Because you physically make it seem like that note is extremely challenging to sing, and your voice's volume matches the previous belting notes, the "mix-like-belt" note doesn't sound noticeably different to your listeners, which is the goal. In terms of vocal health, you don't sing a pitch in a way that compromises your voice, and you don't sing in a way that compromises your style and sound by using a less-than-impressive "stunt double."

I once auditioned for the regional premiere of a new musical and the composer/lyricist team held the audition. I got called back for the character who has a huge, belty number in the show, which I'd researched and learned in advance. At the callback, when the team "taught me" the song, I chose to sing it in a "mix-like-belt" so I would not knock them over with my big belt when I was supposed to be learning the song. When they were done with the instruction, they looked at each other and said, "Well, it looks like we have another belter on our hands!!" I wanted them to hear me ACTUALLY belt the number, so I corrected them, announcing, "Oh, that wasn't my belt. I am planning to belt it for you." They looked at me with huge, stunned eyes and told me to go for it. I sang it in my belt, and they cast me in the role without hesitation. That is how convincing this little vocal sleight of hand trick can be, and another example of how versatile the mix technique is.

There is a whole chapter devoted to how all this applies to your speaking voice, so I want you to know that even if you're not a singer, knowing whether you place your sound in your chest, your sinus cavities, or your nasal passage does still apply to you, so I want you to understand it. I'll be talking about it in detail in the speaking chapter, so know that your time is coming! And singers, you don't get to skip the speaking chapter because, even if you implement everything you learn in the singing chapters, if you don't also practice vocal health in your speaking, you could still experience vocal fatigue or lose your voice.

PART II

THE BULLSHIT BREAKDOWN

I have to confess that I've been itching to share this particular section of The Bullshit Breakdown ever since I decided to write this book. The various techniques you just learned in Part II probably raised a lot of questions for you, and I won't be surprised at all if it also ruffled some feathers. I've grown very accustomed to that reaction in my teaching and coaching. But I'd like to take a moment to bring up some of the misinformation I'm certain you've heard about placement of your sound and then break down for you why it is complete and utter bullshit.

BELTING

Let's be honest: belting gets a bad rap in the singing world, particularly among strictly classical singers and teachers. I'd like to begin with a list of the things belting is NOT, since you have an entire chapter already defining what it IS.

Belting is NOT:

- Bad for you
- Singing in your chest voice
- A word to describe loud singing
- Mixing
- Achieved with a huge space in the back of your throat
- Painful

The primary reason people believe all this bullshit about belting is that they don't really understand what belting IS. I can extend some grace to them because their concern is that it's going to lead to vocal health issues. But the reason they believe that belting is bad is that singers and teachers typically are unable to distinguish the difference between a belt voice and a chest voice. This inability to discern the difference is really the root of the idea that belting is "bad."

Imagine a person who is unaware that a squirt gun is different from a handgun. If you hold a squirt gun, this unaware person feels terrified and begs you to put down the gun. No amount of explaining that it's just a squirt gun with water in it seems to be able to penetrate their firm belief that it is just as dangerous as a handgun. This person is not unintelligent, they've just never learned about squirt guns. All they have to go on is the fact that both guns look similar in shape and function, and that both are aimed at another person or object with the intent to shoot it.

With singing, because classical technique reigns supreme as the most widely taught technique, often taught as the ONLY technique, the vocabulary doesn't seem to exist to explain what belting actually is or does. So, singers and teachers alike use the only technique and terminology they know, which isn't equipped to properly or safely explain belting.

They recognize that belt and chest are big, booming sounds. They recognize that belt and chest are easier in the lower parts of the range.

These commonalities are what cause unaware singers and teachers to believe belt and chest are one in the same when in fact, they are vastly different from each other – almost completely opposite. The chest voice is a booming sound created with a raised soft palate that can only go so high before having to switch into a head voice. The belt voice is a booming sound created with a neutral soft palate and a calling voice that has no breaks and almost no limits to how high it can go.

The #1 bullshit belief about belting is that it's going to harm your voice, when in fact, it's singing in your classical chest voice past its limit that is bad for you. Yet that misinformation is what is widely taught, which leads to many of the remaining bullshit items on my list.

If people believe that belting is the same as singing in their chest voice, they will conclude that belting is painful and dangerous. Singing out of range with the chest voice is definitely bad and painful for you but this fact about the chest voice does not apply to belting, so when this fact is used to describe belting, it is bullshit.

Because many teachers believe belting is bad for you, they will often teach mixing but refer to it as belting. Belt and mix are both contemporary techniques that are placed in the nose, and both have no breaks, but belt uses a calling voice and mix is effortless. There is a whole swath of singing teachers claiming that they teach belting when, in fact, they teach singers to "cheat" on purpose. This happens because of two reasons: 1) there isn't a lot of accurate information available to explain what belt and mix actually are, and 2) a lot of teachers are afraid of belting because they equate it with singing in a chest voice past its limit. Because mix is fairly effortless, it doesn't seem dangerous. Plus, it sounds very similar to belt, only without all the potential risk.

Singers and teachers who don't fully understand belt often claim that singing in a high belt requires more space in the back of the throat. You learned that this advice is false because when you open up the space in the back of your throat, you are no longer belting. You are using the classical chest voice. Once again, belting is accused of being the same as the chest voice, when they couldn't be any more different.

Belting is often thought of as just loud singing. This idea is only partially bullshit. Belting IS loud singing, but it's just not the name for ALL loud singing. Using the expression "belt it out" to encourage singers to sing loudly is what inspires this misleading piece of bullshit. Belting is loud, but not all loud singing is belting.

THE MIXED REGISTER/MIXED VOICE

WARNING: this piece of bullshit gets me riled up.

In some faraway magical kingdom of fairies and unicorns exists a place where singers are capable of singing in two places at the same time – in two registers of the voice at the same time. Sounds like some wacky voodoo, right? The "mixed voice" often refers to combining a bit of the classical chest voice with a bit of the classical head voice.

I've always wanted to meet someone in person who teaches this particular element of bullshit because I'm dying to ask them to demonstrate for me how it's done.

Remember, the classical technique is made up of the chest voice and the head voice and there is a break in the voice between them.

When I ride my bike and try to shift gears, the bike doesn't have the ability to be in two gears at the same time. If it gets stuck between the two while trying to shift, the bike will just stop. It can't operate if a single gear hasn't been selected. The same with a car. I never learned to drive a stick shift, but I know I can't put the car in a little bit of 2nd gear and a little bit of 3rd gear at the same time. I have to pick one or the other.

Guess what? This concept is the SAME for singing. Think of your head voice and your chest voice as different "gears" for your classical singing. It's physically impossible to be in both "gears" at the same time. A decision has to be made about which voice to sing in. Therefore, this "mixed voice" is complete bullshit.

BREAKS

There is this wacky bullshit myth out there that everyone has a different place in their voice where a break occurs. This idea is total bullshit!! These breaks only exist in the classical technique, so classical singers are the only ones who even need to know this information. For males, the break between the chest voice and the head voice is the F# above middle C. For females, the break between the chest voice and the head voice is the A above middle C. The end.

Okay, maybe not quite the end. Some people DO have different breaks than that, but they are typically the people who believe that singing in a chest voice is the same as belting. They have different breaks in their voices because they have trained the voice to stretch past its limit. This expansion IS possible, but it is one of the quickest ways to experience vocal damage of all kinds. The voice is not designed to go past these limits, and when it does, it suffers the consequences.

Furthermore, there are voice teachers who claim to teach contemporary singing but who refer to the chest voice, the head voice, and the breaks in the voice when doing so, all of which only apply to classical singing. So, if you want to learn how to sing contemporary music, don't be fooled by these charlatans claiming to teach contemporary with a classical vocabulary. Again, they don't try to mislead, it's just that they don't know any better. When the only tool in your toolbox is a hammer, you learn how to use it in other ways. Teachers who only have classical training don't realize there's a whole world outside of classical technique, so they use what they have. And sadly, they end up causing a lot of harm to the singers they teach.

You'll also hear a lot of advice about needing to learn how to smooth through the breaks to make them go away. I have possibly heartbreaking news for you: they'll never go away. You CAN strengthen both sides of them, and as a classical singer, you will want to so you can minimize any weaknesses in your range. But as a contemporary singer, this information is useless because it makes no sense to sing contemporary music using a classical technique.

The mix technique in contemporary singing is dependent upon the strength of your classical technique, though, so I do recommend singing in a classical technique using vocal exercises, but only for the purpose of bringing more strength to the mix voice.

I wish it were not the case, but there is A LOT of bullshit available about singing and vocal health. Just as important as knowing how to never lose your voice again is knowing how to distinguish the truth from the bullshit. When you're ready to take the next steps toward uncovering ALL the bullshit and never losing your voice again, I'd love to talk to you about working with me to achieve your goals. Visit my calendar here to set up a time: **www.getmypowerup.com**.

PART III

SHAPE

HIGH-POWERED HIGH NOTES

CHAPTER 9

PUMP UP THE VOLUME, DANCE

"I think of music as fuel, its spectrum of energy governed by tempi, volume, and heart."

– Twyla Tharp

I learned to dance really late in life for someone who desired to be in professional musical theatre. College was the first time I took dance classes but most everyone in my classes had taken dance since early childhood. Much like vocal technique, I didn't pick up on choreography very quickly or very easily. Unlike singing, I didn't have a natural ability for dance, so I became self-conscious about my weaknesses with dance and those weaknesses fueled my insecurity.

I was in a show once where the choreographer wanted us all to dance full-out so he could see the weak spots in our dancing. He instructed us to be big and animated so if we made a mistake, we made a big, obvious mistake. I was horrified by this request. The last thing I wanted to do was draw attention to my mistakes, and I knew there would be MANY.

When we feel insecure about something, it's not our instinct to approach it with boldness. We tend to hold back and play small in hopes that no one will notice our weaknesses.

When it comes to high notes, it's normal for singers to feel a little afraid to approach them because they feel uncertain and scary. So, it's also natural to hold back a little when it comes time to sing these high notes. The problem with this approach, however, is that high notes require more volume than lower notes. Depending on how high the pitch is, a singer can feel soreness in the throat from not singing the pitch loudly enough. This soreness from lack of volume occurs in all three vocal techniques.

My client, Julie, had the most brilliant realization when she learned to belt. Julie came to me having studied classical singing for many years and she wanted to learn to belt. But, like me, she was hesitant at first because she didn't want to cause damage to her voice from this big, bold singing. As we did exercises at the piano, I could see her trepidation growing the higher we belted.

We got to a pitch that scared her too much to try. She laughed nervously and then professed, "I can't do that one. It's too high!" She looked at me, pleading to prove her wrong. So, I told her she definitely could do it, but she needed to increase her volume so the pitch could come out without scratching her throat. Again, she laughed nervously, confused about how being louder was the answer when she was obviously afraid of singing that high at all. Fear won out and she "cheated" by mixing unintentionally instead of belting the note with more volume. When she cheated, it caused the note to sound wimpy. While she wasn't in danger of hurting her voice by cheating, I wanted her to know she could belt it without hurting her voice – to stop being afraid of belting high.

After continuing to attempt the high belting technique and continuing to "cheat," I explained to Julie that without an increase in volume, not only would it be more difficult for her to execute the high pitch, but the more likely she would hurt her throat. She was straining her cords by singing without the required volume.

That guidance finally resonated with her. She took a firmer stance and a bigger breath. I could see the determination in her eyes. She committed to making more volume and BAM! Her belt came flowing out beautifully. Julie exclaimed, "WOW! You know, belting is like a giant middle finger to your nerves! I realize that the choice I have is either to belt or to be nervous. It's impossible to be both at the same time!"

That little truth bomb is the best reasoning I've heard for the need for more volume. Julie realized that her fear held her back physically, and it held back her volume. By holding back in these two ways, she made it impossible to sing the high note correctly. The only choice she had if she wanted to sing the high note correctly was to release her fear about being louder and just do it anyway. When she made the decision to let go of her fear, she was able to belt correctly. And boy, was it stunning!

Whether you are singing classical music or contemporary, whether you are singing in classical, in belt, or in mix, when the pitches start getting higher, the way to make them come out safely is to increase your volume. No matter how scary it may seem to sing high notes really loudly when you feel uncertain, it's the only solution unless you wish to compromise your vocal health. High belting requires more volume to avoid strain. I don't like to recommend mixing or even using Mix Like Belt as a solution to fear, but those are other safe options.

This is a good place to remind you that body awareness is crucial to preventing voice loss and fatigue. Additionally, EACH of the steps in this book must be followed simultaneously in order to prevent vocal damage. On their own they are fabulous additions to your singing, but when used together as directed, they are the key to staying vocally healthy at all times.

Being loud can be scary in general. Doing something already scary and doing it LOUDER can feel paralyzing. Just like I was afraid to dance bigger so I could boldly make a mistake, Julie was afraid to sing bigger so she could boldly make a mistake. In her case, though, singing louder was less about discovering mistakes and more about allowing the high pitch to come out safely and correctly without pain.

If there's a pitch in a song you've been struggling to sing because it feels too high for you, commit to trying it out today or tomorrow with the promise that you will belt loudly, no matter how scary it seems. When you COMMIT to the decision to be louder, you increase the likelihood that you'll succeed!

CHAPTER 10

WIDE OPEN SPACES

"Because things grow. Wherever there is air and light and open space, things grow."

– Helen Oyeyemi

I used to travel full-time with my ex-husband for his work. We were in a different city almost every week, which meant a life of packing, unpacking, and adjusting to a new environment. Some people who experience this lifestyle just live out of their suitcases, but I couldn't do that. Even though we typically spent only seven days in each city, I still wanted it to feel like home. I didn't want to feel like I was always on the run or like I had no place to call home. My goal was to make sure each place we ended up felt like home.

Sometimes we stayed in hotels, other times we got condos or houses on Airbnb. Some of our "homes" were very small and others were quite spacious. There were two lessons I learned during this time in my life: 1) no matter the size, with a little creativity, ANY room can be transformed into enough space, and 2) the more space I had available to me, the more comfortable my temporary home felt, and the more productive I was able to be in the week.

I bet the hotels I stayed in thought I was high maintenance. If I got to the room and it had unnecessary furniture in it, I asked them to remove it. And I always "remodeled" the space. I rearranged everything that wasn't bolted to the floor so that it would flow better for my needs that week.

I traveled with Command hooks because it was always surprising to me how many hotels had ONE towel bar even though they supplied us with three or four sets of towels each day. What if I needed all four of those towels? Where was I supposed to hang the other three? I traveled with power strips because there were rarely enough outlets to function. I brought my own hangers because... well, if you've EVER stayed in a hotel, I'm pretty sure I don't need to explain that one!

Sometimes there were no nightstands. Or there was only one (something my symmetry-demanding brain will never understand). So, we got creative and learned that our big suitcases made perfect makeshift nightstands in a pinch. Plus, this solution provided a place to store the suitcases. The craziest thing I traveled with was a portable kitchen. I had a two-burner induction electric stove and a convection toaster oven, plus all the cookware and bakeware necessary to use them. Those traveled in the big trucks along with my ex's work stuff, and they lived at his work except for the weeks we needed them. I once made an entire Thanksgiving dinner in my hotel room.

I was able to convert ANY space we occupied to meet our needs for the week. Once everything had an appropriate place, the space felt open, clean, and functional – like home.

Space is a pretty magnificent commodity that a lot of people take for granted. I know I did until I started traveling full-time. When it comes to vocal health, space is taken for granted and under-utilized, especially concerning singing high notes.

High notes require added volume, but the other requirement for high notes to come out without causing any strain or scratchy feelings in the throat is space. However, the appropriate shape of space matters. For classical singing, the soft palate is raised like a yawn, so the space needed for high notes requires dropping the jaw as much as possible first. Then, once it's been dropped as low as it can go, we then widen the mouth from the corners like we would if we were to take a bite of a giant burger. So, as you ascend in pitch, your jaw should drop more and more until you reach a pitch that also requires you to widen your mouth a bit. This kind of space required for these high notes is often the one element standing between a singer and her desire to sing a really high pitch.

When you sing in contemporary techniques the soft palate is in its neutral position, and you choose either a belt or a mix, the space needed for high notes is the complete opposite of what is used for classical high notes. With contemporary techniques, you're going to widen your mouth– kind of like a giant, fake smile – as you ascend in pitch as much as much as you can first and then start dropping the jaw.

Without making this necessary space when attempting a high note, you can expect one of two things to happen: 1) the note won't even come out, or 2) it's going to feel scratchy or "pinchy" as I call it. The same is true if you don't increase your volume, actually.

Sometimes, singers do everything else correctly in terms of technique, but they do not make the appropriate space or volume required for the high notes in their songs and they end up with vocal fatigue or voice loss as a result. This issue can be very confusing if you use proper technique otherwise, but correct space is often overlooked.

There's a lot of inconsistent information in the vocal industry about space and "openness" when it comes to singing. It's quite common for singers to end up taking the wrong advice with regard to singing high notes, which can result in all forms of vocal damage.

For example, did you notice that the direction and order the mouth moves to make space for the contemporary techniques is the exact opposite of what it is for classical technique? Since the classical technique seems to be what everyone knows so well, it's very common for a contemporary singer, who might even belt or mix correctly, to hear the *incorrect* advice that they should open up the space in the back of the throat in order to sing their high notes. For classical singing, a space in the back is required. But as we've discussed, if a contemporary singer opens up the space in the back of the throat, they will no longer be singing in a contemporary technique. They will instead be singing in a classical technique which is very limiting in regard to staying safe. If the singer attempts a high note as a contemporary singer, then there's no chance that pitch is in the safe zone of the classical chest voice. Opening the space in the back of the throat is extremely dangerous advice. Again, there is no malice intended; it's sadly just ignorance of how the contemporary voice is meant to function. But if the singer follows this advice, they will end up experiencing vocal fatigue and possibly even voice loss.

So, space in the correct location is your FRIEND when it comes to singing high notes beautifully, effortlessly, and without strain or pain. If you want help mastering your high notes, we should chat about a coaching program that would be the best fit for you. You can schedule a time to chat with me here: **www.getmypowerup.com**.

CHAPTER 11

A CHANGE WOULD DO YOU GOOD

"The secret of change is to focus all your energy not on fighting the old but on building the new."

- Socrates

I like to talk to myself. Out loud. And I work from home by myself so it's something I do unabashedly and frequently. I once found myself in a grocery store talking out loud to myself, and I kept trying to lower my volume so no one would hear me. However, I'm certain everyone could still see my mouth moving. One of the cool things about wearing masks during the pandemic was that I could talk to myself out loud, and no one would know. But before that, it was a struggle.

So, I taught myself ventriloquism.

There are two lessons to be found in this illustration. The first is about altering how we speak and the second about being able to achieve a goal by modifying the way we approach it.

In this part of the book, we talked a lot about high notes and how they have to be treated differently than other pitches in songs. High notes require more volume and space in order to come out both beautifully and healthily. But there's one last piece to this puzzle of healthy and gorgeous high notes: vowel modification.

As we discussed in the last chapter, there are certain directions the mouth must go to allow for a high pitch to be produced without causing strain or pain to the vocal cords. With classical, there is space in the back of the throat, so the jaw drops all the way before beginning to widen the mouth for high notes. With contemporary, there is no space in the back of the throat and the mouth is widened as far as it can go before dropping the jaw to produce a high note.

But imagine the high note of a contemporary song is on the word "know." In a contemporary song, we widen the mouth first before dropping the jaw, but an "oh" vowel causes the mouth to round as if blowing through a straw. A rounded mouth that is fairly closed isn't going to be able to accommodate a high pitch, so in this instance, the vowel must be modified.

Because high notes require more space that must take on a specific shape depending on which technique is being used, there are specific vowels that are tricky for high pitches. These vowels challenge the ability to make this space and shape simultaneously. The answer is NOT to change the technique being used, but instead to change the shape of the vowel.

When I learned ventriloquism, the same theory applied. Most vowels and consonants could be produced with my lips slightly separated and making a sort of fake smile. But certain sounds – both vowels and consonants – needed modification. In ventriloquism, you don't want your lips to be visibly moving, so any sounds that would normally cause a lip movement need to be modified. For example, an "mm" produced the traditional way requires both lips to come together while making sound. In ventriloquism, that action is visible, so instead we place the tongue on the roof of the mouth right behind the upper front teeth and flatten the tip just a bit so more of the tongue touches the roof of the mouth.

Say "mom" with the "m" in this position. It's kind of like an "n", and then you add a small, subtle "uh" at the end, almost like "NAWN(uh)", and it somehow sounds like "mom." With ventriloquism, the mouth makes small adjustments to the way sound is produced, but the ear of the listener still hears the word that is intended.

The same principle is true for vowel modification in singing. In classical singing, the jaw is dropped before it widens, but also the lips make what I call a "soft pucker" in order to properly shape the vowels. Pucker up like you're about to kiss someone but then release the pucker a bit so your lips are soft. In this position, say these vowel sound: Maw, Meh, Moh, Moo. Now, say "moo" again, but this time allow your tongue to make a "mee" vowel inside the shape of "moo". I call this "an E through an OOH," and it is the correct way to pronounce E vowels in classical singing.

The easiest way to remember how to modify most classical shapes is to think of the yawn space. Have you ever had a yawn interrupt what you are saying? It's very challenging to understand what someone is saying when they are simultaneously yawning and speaking. Singing while yawning is the best description I have for how it feels to properly sing vowels in a classical shape.

When we move into contemporary singing, because the mouth is widened and then dropped, there are different vowels that are tricky. In contemporary singing, the vowels are shaped just like they are when we speak. If we are singing a high pitch on the word "know" in either a belt or a mix, because the vowel is an "oh" sound, it causes our mouth to close around into a small circle which doesn't lend itself to a widened mouth. The tricky vowel "oh" in this instance needs to be modified to an easier shape so the high note has the required space to come out. In this case, I recommend singing the "oh" vowel as if you are someone with a Southern accent. In the South, an "oh" vowel typically has a little bit of an "eh" and an "ooh" in front of it, like "ehh-ooh-oh." When you make the first two vowel sounds before the "oh" in this example, it forces your mouth to widen, which is exactly what we want, and the listeners hear the word "know," just like we intended. Their brains automatically piece together the logical best choice for what that word could be instead of noticing the odd pronunciation.

So, in contemporary singing, the tricky vowels are the ones which require the mouth to be more closed. We modify tricky vowels to be shapes that allow a widening of the vowels.

There is a contemporary song I love to sing in a mix technique, and the word "world" is one of the highest notes in the song. If I pronounce "world" the same way I do when I speak the word, it sounds horrible in the song, and it is very challenging to sing the correct pitch. My mouth doesn't make enough space for a healthy vowel to be produced because my lips round for the "whir" sound, then my tongue gets in the way for the "RLD", leaving not much room in my mouth to produce a high note. So, in this case, I use a British pronunciation of "world" (more like "wuhld") which gives the vowel exactly what it needs – more space without lifting in the back – and it allows my listeners to be able to identify the correct word.

In contemporary singing, I like to call the required space "mouth space" so it doesn't get confused with an "open space" like in classical. Mouth space is everything forward of the molars; open space is everything behind them.

With my clients, I offer a "Vowel Modification Cheat Sheet" to help them modify their tricky vowels easier. If you'd like to grab a copy of that cheat sheet, you can do so here:

www.singwithoutlimits.com/vowelmodificati on.

PART III

THE BULLSHIT BREAKDOWN

Ahhh... I don't think I knew how much I needed this outlet for expressing my frustration with the myths and lies this industry perpetuates. I'm sure you can imagine how aggravating it has been the past two decades to constantly argue and defend my evidence for voice-loss prevention against all the bullshit. Or how aggravating it is that the bullshit never seems to go away. This misinformation is the reason I wanted to write this book.

I'm not just looking for an outlet to vent, I want the face of the music industry to transform. I want it to be abnormal for a singer, actor, or public speaker to lose their voice. I want it to be unheard of that a performer should hear from any kind of instructor or coach that voice loss is something they should expect to experience, like having a cold. I want it to be extremely rare that a performer ever needs to cancel a series of gigs because of vocal damage. So, I can't just tell you how to do something, I also have to tell you what's wrong with the way you've done it or what you believed about it.

Part III is all about shape and its role in vocal health, particularly as it relates to high notes. Some of my favorite nuggets of bullshit surrounding this topic can be found in this chapter. Are you ready to break it all down? Let's do it!

I'M AN ALTO (No, you're not)

Honestly, I wish so very much that we could just end this particular discussion right there with the section title, but I already know there are several of you clutching your pearls at the thought of me suggesting you aren't altos. So, I'll explain why I'm not only suggesting that you're not an alto, I'm insisting it.

It's actually very rare to be a true alto. And I'm NOT TALKING ABOUT IN CHOIR. I sang alto in my high school and college choirs as well as in a professional choir and I'm most definitely a soprano. You more than likely are as well. In choir, I like to think of your "part" as your "voice assignment" because typically, the treble section of a choir is filled with sopranos who are divided among the different voice parts, so each section has enough voices.

How do you know what part you really are then if your assignment in choir wasn't the right answer? For starters, your voice part is based on the timbre of your voice, not your range. In other words, range isn't what separates singers into voice parts, contrary to what you've likely been told or been led to believe.

A soprano and a mezzo soprano technically have the same vocal range. I know you don't believe me but hear me out. A mezzo soprano has a darker timbre to her voice. Her voice is richer, fuller, and darker which, to the untrained ear, can be mistaken for sounding lower in pitch when it's not lower at all. A soprano has a lighter, often brighter sound which, again, can be mistaken for sounding higher in pitch when it's not. A mezzo and a soprano singing the same exact pitch will sound very different. THAT difference is what makes one a mezzo and the other a soprano.

Altos, however, are extremely rare. Their sound is so dark and so rich that these voices are often mistaken for men. Yet, altos have the same range as sopranos and mezzo-sopranos. I can feel you arguing with me through the pages, but it's true. ALL females have the same vocal range; it's the timbre of the voice that distinguishes a soprano from a mezzo from an alto, NOT the range.

I always give the examples of Tracy Chapman and Nina Simone who have true alto voices. They spent their lives being confused for men because of the dark, rich timbre of their voices which causes the ear to think they are speaking or singing lower than they are. But sing a line of one of Tracy Chapman's songs, and you'll notice right away that, even though you're singing in the same octave she is, she sounds like she's singing lower than you are. You are both able to sing the same notes with the same ease, but she sounds dramatically different than you do.

In a choir, the darkest voices work the best in the alto section – not because of range, but because the weight of their voices carries the lower pitches more beautifully. Likewise, the sopranos work the best on the top line because the lightness of their voices sounds effortless and dexterous which is perfect for the highest pitches. The mezzos are perfect for filling out the middle because their darkness is meatier than the sopranos but lighter than the altos, making for a perfectly balanced, rounded, and complete sound in the treble section.

Unfortunately, most of the time, choirs are full of sopranos and mezzo-sopranos who are assigned to a part whether or not it suits their voices. While I'm most definitely a soprano, I sang alto in choir because I can read music, I'm confident in my singing and am not afraid to sing out, and because I can hear harmonies really well. NOT because I am actually an alto, because I'm definitely not.

My voice teacher begged my high school choir director to let me sing soprano because she wanted me to exercise my full vocal range rather than hang out in the vocal basement all the time. He made a compromise and put me in the second soprano section because that part also requires a good music reader and a good ear, since the harmonies are in the middle. He didn't want to waste my reading and listening skills on the melody when he could use singers on the melody who didn't excel at other elements of singing. And THAT example is why your voice assignment from choir is likely irrelevant when it comes to defining your voice.

Also, most of the singing population believes they have a limited vocal range. Choir directors and voice teachers aren't doing much of anything to dispel this myth. Because singers and teachers alike believe that their ranges are limited, the singer is thrown into the alto section because of a mistaken belief that they can't sing high notes.

You might think that I've lost my mind at this point. Whenever I explain this viewpoint to a group of singers, there is ALWAYS at least one person who shakes her head, saying I just don't understand her and that it's different for her – she really CAN'T sing high notes. I always reassure these confident liars that they CAN in fact sing these high notes. They just haven't yet learned how.

Which brings me to my next piece of bullshit:

INCREASING YOUR RANGE

I admit I have put out ads offering the ability to increase your range even though I know it's total bullshit. I've done it because the vast majority of the singing population believes it's possible to increase their range and they are actively looking for a way to do it. I simply show them how to access the range they already have but didn't know how to reach without instruction.

Here's the truth about your range: it exists in its entirety from the moment you are born, you just don't know how to access all of it until you're shown how. But it's all there right now. So, when singers tell me they "CAN'T" sing high notes, I call bullshit. I know they can and, typically, I prove it to them in a matter of moments. Let me explain with an example:

I HATE working out. When my husband first left me, the FIRST thing I did (after taking down all our photos together and throwing them in the trash) was cancel my gym membership. It was the biggest waste of $20/month I'd ever spent because I hated going and would come up with every reason under the sun not to go. And yes, I KNOW I have to do some kind of physical movement for my health, but the gym is NOT how I choose to do it.

You see, I have to be tricked into exercising which is impossible at the gym. If I go for a gorgeous hike, there's not only a massive benefit to my health from the hike, but there's often a reward at the end: a beautiful view. And just like that, I tricked myself into doing exercise. If I take a salsa dancing class, in no time I'm sweating my brains out, my quads are quivering, and my heart is pumping. I feel like a sexy and flirtatious goddess. But look at that, once again, I managed to trick myself into exercising.

Knowing this inclination about myself, I harnessed that same magic to help singers who stubbornly insisted they were altos because they "couldn't sing high notes." I helped them trick themselves into singing into the stratosphere with ease. They all sang their full three-octave range without any strain the very first time I asked them to do it. I just tricked them into it by making the process so easy, they didn't even know how high they were singing until I pointed it out. And the reward was that they broke through a limitation in their singing, realizing they actually CAN sing high notes. It's not even that hard to do.

We learned the tricks of how to sing high notes effectively and without strain in Part III because this limitation is a frequent cause of vocal damage of all kinds. It's also a limitation that has no logical reason to exist.

The other main piece of bullshit about range is that everyone's range is different. BULLSHIT. It's not. If you're a female, you have the same range as every other female, which is three octaves at Eb. Some singers learn how to access notes beyond their three octaves in each direction, but every female has the same three octaves available to her. Also, you have the same breaks in your voice as every other female.

As for males, I'm still working on my theory here, but I'm starting to believe the same is true for males as it is for females – that every male has the same range, but it is timbre, not range, that determines whether they are a tenor or a baritone or a bass. I'm not yet willing to state that idea unequivocally, but it's a theory I'm still trying to prove.

OPEN THROAT

This mistruth is without a doubt my favorite piece of bullshit. I once made a graphic that was like a Brady Bunch image of screenshots of various voice teachers on YouTube explaining the need for an "open throat" or "open sound" or "open space" when singing high notes. They were all contemporary teachers.

By now you recognize that an "open" anything related to space in the throat refers to classical singing. Either that, or it refers to how to destroy your voice singing contemporary music in a chest voice. However, the bulk of what is taught in the industry is that you need to create more space in the back of your throat to sing high notes in your contemporary singing. Once again, this practice is probably the fastest way possible to damage your voice. Yet, it's widely taught because classical technique is the only vocabulary available for singers, even though it is the complete opposite of what is needed to sing contemporary music.

Now that you've learned you're (more than likely) NOT an alto and that your true voice part has nothing to do with your range (which is HUGE!), I hope you're eager to learn how to access your entire range with ease like my clients have who started out right where you are. When learning to access your full range, the difference between open space and mouth space can literally save your voice when it comes to shaping high notes. The kind of shape you make with your mouth to accommodate high notes all comes down to whether you are a classical singer or a contemporary singer, which of course is defined by the position of your soft palate.

If you are ready to take the next steps toward accessing your full range with ease, I'd love to talk with you about working together. You can set up a time to talk with me here:

www.getmypowerup.com.

PART IV

CONSISTENCY

POWERFUL HABITS FOR CONSISTENT HEALTH

CHAPTER 13

SILENCE SPEAKS A THOUSAND WORDS

"Only one thing is more frightening than speaking your truth, and that is not speaking."

– Naomi Wolf

Tonight, I'm making risotto for dinner. I learned how to make it almost 20 years ago and it's one of my standard, go-to, easy dishes that I love to make. One of my favorite things about risotto is that I can put anything in it that I have on hand, and the instructions for making it are virtually the same. There is a basic recipe or formula for making the base meal, and then you can cook up literally anything else you want to add to it.

This versatility of risotto is also present in my vocal method. We've talked at length about how to use the method for singing, and you can follow the very same formula for speaking. In this chapter, I'll "translate" for you how to apply each of the components of what you've learned to your speaking voice.

Not only can you follow the same formula for speaking as you do for singing, but if you only follow the protocol for singing and don't also apply it to your speaking, you will still be at risk for vocal damage.

In Part I, we talked about establishing your foundation which is made up of breath, support, and connection. As a speaker (or during the speaking portions of your life), this same foundation is required to stay vocally healthy.

First, just like with your singing, you will want to make sure you are always taking in a relaxed, low breath. I typically recommend practicing this type of breathing when you are doing something mindless, like driving somewhere you are familiar with. Draw your attention to your belly and see if you are able to take in a low breath before speaking.

As we discussed earlier, it is very natural for us to breathe correctly when not thinking about it. But when we draw our attention to our breath, our overthinking brains kick in and try to disrupt nature. Being as relaxed as possible is key to successful low breathing because it allows nature to take the front seat rather than your brain, which will try to manipulate your breath every single time.

If you practice low breathing in your car, repeating the text of the commercials you hear on the radio, for example, is a great way to speak on a low breath. While you're at it, initiate the sound of this repeated radio commercial text with your core abdominal muscles with a tuck of support. Even though it seems like making the tuck will expel your air faster, it actually does the opposite – it prolongs it, so you have plenty of air to get through your whole thought.

Something to note about the support process is that you can create the tucking motion of your core abdominal muscles with or without breath. I often ask clients to practice this motion without breath so they can get used to utilizing the muscles. Just like you might quickly tuck in your belly as someone snaps a photo of you, without involving your breath in it at all, the same is possible for you in your speaking and singing. This possibility allows you to practice tucking separately from breathing, but it is also why some people end up holding their breath. If you notice that you exhale extra air at the end of each thought, ensure that you aren't holding your breath by fluttering your lips like a motorboat with a low breath and a tuck of your belly muscles. If you can accomplish this task, you are successfully connecting your sound to your breath.

Work on incorporating your foundation into your speaking as your first step toward speaking with vocal health. Your foundation is the most important piece of the puzzle with speaking. Once you have your breath, support, and connection committed to muscle memory in your speaking, you can move on to the other elements.

Once I started making my foundation a normal part of creating sound of any kind, it became challenging for me to NOT utilize my foundation. Sometimes when I work with clients, I like to demonstrate the difference between making sound properly vs. making sound improperly with regard to foundation. I have to really concentrate in order to make sound without a low breath or without tucking in my abdominal muscles. That's how committed to muscle memory this foundation is for me. You for it to become such a regular part of how you make sound that you have to think really hard about it to do it incorrectly.

I will say that foundation – particularly the support element of it – is often the missing piece for singers and speakers alike in their abilities to prevent voice loss. So, I can't recommend enough that you practice this until it becomes part of your muscle memory.

In Part II, we learned about having the appropriate placement for each style of music you sing. Just like with contemporary singing, there is very little need for classical placement when it comes to speaking. As a reminder, classical placement refers to having a raised soft palate that blocks off the passageway into the nose.

For all of you actors, I know you have likely been taught that this is exactly the kind of space you need to be making in your mouth as often as is possible. I was taught the same information when I was in acting programs. However, just like how your chest voice has a limit in your singing, that limit still exists in your speaking voice. If you lift your palate, you will be speaking in your chest voice and will need to be very conscious of the pitch of your speaking voice, especially if you have to project your speaking, so that you won't stretch your voice past its limit.

Instead, I suggest that you speak in more of a belt placement which makes the range limitations go away since there are no breaks or needs to shift your sound into a different place in your body. Most people innately speak in a belt placement often without even being aware of it. I have met people – usually women – who speak in a mix as opposed to a belt, which I find interesting because it isn't as common. Speaking in a mix is a much softer, lighter way to speak.

We all speak a certain way by default. In order to stay vocally healthy, you must identify what your "default voice" is with regard to vocal placement. Once you know what your default voice tends to be, you will know how to best apply my vocal method to your speaking voice to stay healthy consistently. But keep in mind, even with practice, your vocal technique can morph into something different when you are on stage in any capacity because nerves and adrenaline are added to the mix. Developing muscle memory AND body awareness is so vital to staying healthy.

For example, you may discover that you tend to speak in a classical placement. Your voice may sound booming, dark, and somewhat stuffy or proper sounding. It's quite common for actors – particularly classical stage actors – to speak in this placement by default, at least when on a stage. If you discover this placement for your stage voice, you can practice moving that open, classical chest voice into a belt which is much healthier and will allow you way more range while keeping the power of your sound. Remember that the belt voice doesn't have any breaks in it, nor does it have any danger zones or limitations on how high you can take it. This is why belt is the best choice for speaking powerfully.

The way to work on this technique is to practice speaking in a baby belt first – with your voice really forward with a scrunched-up nose and a widened mouth – until you are confident that you consistently speak in that placement, instead of lifting in the back and placing sound in your chest.

I once had a side-hustle as the head of merchandise for the National Tour of the Broadway play, "The Curious Incident of the Dog in the Night-time." This play was almost three hours long and chock-full of yelling and screaming. The actors frequently felt fatigued and lost their voices which pained me GREATLY, since I knew exactly why it happened.

While out at a speakeasy one night with a few of the actors and technicians, I got into a conversation about how making a small shift in vocal placement could eliminate vocal fatigue. One of the actors pulled me aside and asked more questions, curious about if what I proposed was possible for her. I agreed to teach her this small little tip in exchange for letting me record her feedback about using my tip in her performance.

Her experience was very powerful. She performed in eight shows per week and required a LOT of yelling in her roles. Yet instead of feeling exhausted and having to put herself on vocal rest until she had to perform again, she felt energized after her shows – even on days when she had two shows. She didn't even learn ALL of my steps, just the placement piece. The only element we changed was lowering her soft palate to the neutral position, so she placed her sound forward in a belt instead of in an open, classical placement. She learned that she had been using her chest voice, so any time she had to yell, she pushed her chest voice higher than it was meant to go. When she belted instead, projecting was effortless and painless for her. She was able to speak her lines with just as much power but without the strain from before. Oftentimes, the elements of Part II and Part III can blend together, and Charlotte's experience is a perfect example of that fact.

You can hear Charlotte's story by visiting this link: **www.singwithoutlimits.com/charlotte**

In Part III, we learned about shape, particularly with regard to high notes. When speaking, however, we don't have a piano or a pitch pipe handy to identify the pitches we use to speak. So, knowing whether we are in the danger zone when speaking in a classical placement can be really tricky since the limitations on the chest voice still exist as well as the breaks between chest and head. Just like with singing, one of the main reasons I recommend using a belt placement instead is because it doesn't have the limitations of the classical placement. When it comes to speaking, an increase in pitch often comes with increased volume. Because of this correlation, if you tend to speak in a classical placement – with a lot of space in the back of the throat – you are likely to wear out quickly, especially if you have to speak with considerable volume.

If you notice that you experience fatigue after speaking at a higher volume than normal, in addition to making sure that you speak in a belt placement instead of a classical one, make sure that you create mouth space (space in the mouth forward of the molars) in the appropriate direction to accommodate the potentially rising pitch of your voice. When belting, we want to widen our mouths prior to lowering the jaw. Use the same rule of thumb for speaking as for singing. If you have to yell, make sure you widen your vowel shapes as you project so that you allow the pitch and volume of your voice enough space in your mouth. Avoid lifting in the back of the throat which will shift you into a classical placement and put you at risk for vocal damage.

The kind of mouth space you want should exist only from your molars forward.

Just like with singing, if all three of these components don't work together in your speaking, you put yourself at risk for damaging your voice. Practice foundation first, then once you've mastered it, move on to make sure your placement is correct, and finally ensure that you create the appropriate shapes and amount of space to accommodate high volume and an increase in pitch.

Singers, make sure you practice these same steps in your singing AND in your speaking so you can permanently prevent voice loss and fatigue.

CHAPTER 14

YOU GOT THE RIGHT STUFF, BABY

"Either you run the day, or it runs you."

– Jim Rohn

I'm not a creature of habit. I've been an entrepreneur my entire life and, with the exception of grade school and high school, I've never had a schedule where I got up at the same time every day.

As an adult who is completely in charge of my entire schedule and responsibilities, I've often wished that routine and habit were part of my life because it can make me feel like a rudderless scatterbrain at times because no two days look alike. I've (unsuccessfully) attempted at various times to make routine and habit a consistent part of my life. I'm confessing this to you because it feels slightly inauthentic of me to ask you to form daily habits when I am not one to form such routines. However, when it comes to vocal health, I am unusually consistent about having a system for healthy habits.

I love the quote for this chapter. I have no idea who Jim Rohn is, but his words shook me to my core because they are so spot on, particularly for the topic of vocal health. You have learned what to do to stay healthy, but the truth of the matter is that you MUST make the decision every single day to prioritize your vocal health if you want to see a change that permanently prevents voice loss and vocal fatigue. No one is going to hold you to this responsibility. YOU must commit to doing the work.

The advantage my clients have is that I hold them accountable and check in with them on a regular basis to see how they're doing with regard to their performing and vocal health. Accountability makes a humongous difference, but they still have to do the work. I can't do it for them. They still have to put in the practice so they can develop muscle memory, and you will have to do the same.

I'd love to talk with you about what it looks like for me to support you as you embark on your journey to permanently prevent voice loss and vocal fatigue. If you're ready to take the next step, get on my calendar for a conversation by visiting:

www.getmypowerup.com.

Let's shift our focus onto some habits that will supplement all the work you're doing to develop healthy vocal technique and muscle memory. Please note that these things are "supplements" to a healthy voice, NOT replacements for modifying your technique. Most often, I encounter people who only use these kinds of tips and tricks to address vocal fatigue and voice loss once it's already happened. THAT STOPS NOW.

Once you implement the steps of my Unlimited Vocal Health™ System, all the practices listed here will be bonus tips, NOT how you battle voice loss symptoms. Why? Because you will no longer experience voice loss or vocal fatigue once this method is in your body and part of your life.

THERE ARE NO QUICK FIXES FOR VOCAL DAMAGE. PERIOD. If you lose your voice, or you experience vocal fatigue, the ONLY cure to bring back your voice is vocal rest. The tools and tips I'm about to share with you are just supplements, NOT solutions or fixes. And ideally, you will implement what you've learned, so voice loss and vocal fatigue will become a thing of the past.

To download my full list of vocal health dos and don'ts, visit this link:

https://singwithoutlimits.com/vocalhealthtips

I'm going to highlight a few of the most important points in this chapter, but you may want the cheat sheet at the link above to keep as a reference. This link includes the best "dos" for vocal health, the important "don'ts," and the "what to do if you're sick" points.

THE DOs

The most important "dos" for vocal health are the most obvious ones: get plenty of water and rest. Water and rest are your very best friends for staying vocally healthy. Water keeps all of your muscles – vocal and otherwise – hydrated so they stay in top shape. Singing and dehydration are a dangerous combination because the voice needs the hydration only water provides in order to stay lubricated. Drinking water is sort of like keeping enough oil in your car.

Sleep allows your body to recharge – kind of like a mini vocal rest. Sleep also helps your body better utilize the hydration from the water you are drinking. The longer you are awake without sleep, the more your body depletes the resources it has. Interestingly, you can follow the entire method in this book but if you're not getting plenty of sleep and water, you are still at risk for damaging your voice.

I have a client who follows my method to a tee and is a complete powerhouse of a singer, but her work schedule and her "mom schedule" are so demanding that sleep is extremely hard for her to come by. As a result, she suffered from vocal fatigue this past year, even though she's doing everything else correctly. Sleep is ESSENTIAL to staying vocally healthy.

Putting yourself on vocal rest when you are fatigued is extremely important. Again, it is my hope that you will implement what you've learned in this book so that fatigue will no longer be something you experience. But if you aren't able to implement it, or if you end up doing something incorrectly, I want you to promise me you will put yourself on vocal rest to heal. No playing the tough guy and muscling through the fatigue. Trust me, I tried it and can vouch that this "solution" doesn't work.

Vocal rest is reserved for when the damage has already been done. If you lose your voice or if you feel fatigued, vocal rest is the answer. When you put yourself on vocal rest, aim to spend the bulk of your day in silence, but set aside three to four times each day to do some very light humming in various parts of your range. Even better, do your humming in the shower or in a steamy bathroom. The humming will loosen any phlegm that builds up and it helps your vocal cords stay warm, so they don't atrophy while you rest them.

Get as much sleep as you possibly can while on vocal rest. You also need to stay hydrated so your vocal mechanisms can heal. The very best choice for hydration is large quantities of room-temperature water. Singers often complain about the room-temperature" part of that instruction, but I like to remind them that the temperature inside their bodies is quite a bit warmer than the temperature inside their rooms. With that in mind, room temperature water is cold enough. If your drink is too cold, it can lead to tense muscles among other issues. On the flipside of that, if your beverage is still steaming hot, it can also jar your system. When drinking hot beverages, make sure to wait for the steam to go away before consuming them.

As for the quantity of water you need, the traditional rule of thumb is to divide your weight in half. This number is how many ounces of water you need to drink each day. When you are sick, on vocal rest, or using your voice more than normal, I recommend upping your water intake significantly. If you're sick or on vocal rest, hydration is one of the most important parts of the healing process. Keeping hydrated allows your body to flush out what's causing you to feel sick and replenish you with something clean. Being sick depletes your body's hydration and healing happens so much faster when water comes in regularly to flush out the "ick" and keep you lubricated. If you use your voice far more than normal, you will get dehydrated faster, so it's a good idea to proactively drink more water than usual to stay hydrated.

THE DON'Ts

I think I could write endlessly about what not to do, but I don't want to sound like a nagging finger-pointer who's taking away all your fun. Plus, you can download the handout that has all the don'ts spelled out for you. Instead, I'm going to focus on some of the most important ones. I know if I overwhelm you with too many things to stop doing, you won't stop doing ANY of them.

Clearing your throat is one of the worst things you can do to your voice. Typically, when I tell someone how bad it is for them, they feel the need to do it more frequently, so there's your warning. If your throat feels like you need to clear it, doing some low, chesty humming can rid your lungs of the phlegm. Or you can try a little trick I made up that works like magic which I call "silent clearing." I made a quick video that might be helpful which you can check out by visiting: **www.singwithoutlimits.com/silentclearing**.

Try to do the following steps slowly while you figure out how silent clearing works. First, bring together the muscles of your throat as if you were about to clear your throat the usual way, but DON'T ALLOW YOUR VOICE TO MAKE ANY SOUND. Slowly, feel the muscles press together, and then the back of your tongue will feel as though it's clearing something from your throat, so just swallow. That's it. It does the same thing only it isn't trashing your voice from the grinding vocals that usually accompany a throat clearing.

Another significant no-no is whispering. Please don't whisper at all if you can help it. This action is just as hard on your voice as screaming (obviously the unsupported, incorrectly placed kind of screaming). I've encountered many a singer on vocal rest who whispered because she wasn't supposed to talk, blissfully unaware that this choice made her condition worse rather than providing a workaround for not being allowed to speak. Whispering is not just a practice to avoid on vocal rest; it should be avoided all the time.

Here's a don't for when you are sick: please don't take numbing or anesthetizing medicines, drops, teas, or sprays to feel better. These kinds of "cures" just mask your symptoms, so you no longer feel them. Then, when you try to sing while you magically feel better, you end up making the issue worse. Other medicines to avoid unless absolutely necessary are the kinds that dry out your sinuses. Having excess mucous when you are sick is no fun, but these kinds of meds tend to dry out everything, leaving you dehydrated.

I was once scheduled to record an album in a studio and had to take a medicine for clearing excess mucous. I had booked the appointment to record and paid my deposit, but I ended up with a nasty sinus infection the day of recording. I had seven songs to record that day, so I considered this one of those "absolutely necessary" kinds of situations and I took a 12-hr nose spray that cleared out and dried up my sinuses in a matter of seconds. However, because I know it's terrible for my voice to be dried out AND because I had an all-day recording session which would deplete what little hydration I had left, I made sure to drink extra water that day and the few days after my recording session to counteract the medicine.

So, if you find yourself in a situation similar to mine, do what you can to replenish the hydration that is zapped from your body by the dehydrating medicine required to fix the sinus problem.

You can get your own copy of all my vocal health tips here:

https://singwithoutlimits.com/vocalhealthtips

These tips are meant to supplement the changes you'll make to your technique to prevent voice loss and fatigue. They are NOT meant to be a shortcut or a replacement for correcting your technique. On their own, they are not able to keep you vocally healthy, nor are they able to correct any damage you may experience.

To learn more about working with me to prevent voice loss and vocal fatigue for good, visit

www.getmypowerup.com

PART IV

THE BULLSHIT BREAKDOWN

We've talked about how to make the vocal health you learned with your singing voice a consistent part of your daily life by utilizing it with your speaking voice and by implementing some healthy habits to supplement your vocal health practice. Now, it's time to break down the bullshit surrounding this topic, and boy, is there a load of it available.

I recently watched an excruciating video put on by SAG/AFTRA on vocal health for voice actors in the voiceover industry. It featured a panel of people I refuse to call experts who are working voice actors, a speech pathologist, a voice doctor (who didn't get nearly enough time to talk), a voiceover director, and a couple of voice coaches. I took a ton of notes and documented the exact position in the video where they spewed the bullshit which perpetuates all the lies out there about vocal health. It was so painful to watch, I never figured out if I should have laughed or cried.

The bulk of the work that they discussed was about voicing characters for the video game industry. The conversation focused a lot on knowing your limits and setting boundaries with your producers and agents, so the actors could preserve their voices all the way to the end of the recording session.

One of the smelliest piles of bullshit out there is the very focus of that awful video: that there is a limit to the amount of speaking you can do before vocal fatigue and voice loss are inevitable. They perpetuated the notion that there are measures you can take to save your voice and prolong the inevitable as long as possible. Here are some of the bullshit ideas and "tips" that came from this piece of trash:

- When recording multiple characters during a session, strategically order them so you do the most vocally demanding one first because, by the time you get to it at the end, you're not going to have a voice anymore. I also hear this idea from lead singers in bands who strategically order their set lists, so they don't save the big, demanding songs for the end of the gig when they no longer have a voice.

- Tell your producers and directors up front the order you'd like to record and let them know that if you don't go in that order, you won't have enough voice to get through all the scenes in one session. If they insist on going in a different order, leave the gig because it's not worth losing your voice.

- If you are in an ongoing production like a Broadway show and you have a studio recording the same day as one of your performances, make sure you know the limits of what your voice can handle and let them know you have to perform that night so they can work with you to make sure you don't lose your voice before your show.

Some of the bullshit comments everyone involved just took as fact included:

- Four hours of talking will wear out your voice
- Producers know they will not get much from voice actors after two hours of using their voices

Let's break down this bullshit, shall we? Let's begin with the oh-so-NOT-helpful "tips." Armed with all the technique you've learned and implemented from this book, there is no need to devise a gameplan for getting all your work done before losing your voice or getting fatigued. Nor is there any need for you to take charge of your producer's recording plan for you and call the shots as if you're the boss. There is also no need to threaten directors or producers with you walking out on the job if they don't comply with your demands.

Moving on to the bogus "facts." Once again, if you implement what you've learned in this book, you'll be able to work as many hours as the director and producer want you to work, and you can still have enough voice to perform in your Broadway show – twice even – later that same day. You'll be their favorite voice actor because you won't have any of the limitations the other actors come in with.

My 2018 World Champion client was one of the singers in my 2018 vocal health case study which was a five-week study where I walked five singers through my vocal method to prove that it would give singers the ability to never lose their voice again. He participated because he wanted to be able to book wedding gigs which require a minimum of three hours of singing which he wasn't able to do without losing his voice. After the case study, he went on to win a world championship title in an international singing competition.

After he won, he was hired to do some recording in his hometown and his producer asked my client for my contact information because he was so impressed that my client was able to sing full-out for eight hours at a time, multiple days in a row, without experiencing even a little fatigue. My client's producer called to THANK ME for coaching my client and to ask if he could send some of his clients my way so they could have these same superpowers.

That case study and the reprise of it in the spring of 2021 produced some pretty incredible results. If you'd like to check it out, you can do so here: **www.singwithoutlimits.com/vocalhealth**

One of the more interesting comments from that garbage video came from the speech pathologist who shared that in her experience working with American voice actors, most aren't getting enough vocal training. She said that British, Australian, and New Zealander voice actors get far more training than Americans. She added that American actors have a willingness to do whatever the director asks of them, but oftentimes, they sacrifice their own vocal health, likely because they lack proper vocal training.

As a New York City acting conservatory graduate, I can assure you that what I teach in this book was NOT included in my voice acting classes, nor was there any training at all on preventing voice loss or staying vocally healthy. I'm not sure if that kind of training is what the pathologist wished American actors received. Perhaps she was hopeful Americans would gain a better understanding of how to identify their own vocal limitations and define boundaries for what they will and will not do so they can better manage their voice loss and vocal fatigue. Regardless, I agree that performers in general do not receive enough vocal training. In more than two decades of teaching voice (mostly to trained singers and actors), I've never once taught a client who already knew what I have shared with you in this book.

When it comes to maintaining vocal health habits, the bullshit continues to abound plentifully. Here is a short list of the bullshit you will hear (if you haven't already):

- Save your voice for your big event
- This tea, throat spray, lozenge, medicine, beverage, device, essential oil, elixir,

magic potion, witch's spell, handy trick, secret password, etc. will heal your voice

- A personal steamer can heal vocal fatigue
- Marking, the practice of not performing full-out just to rehearse the performance, is recommended to save your voice for the real deal
- Schedule a recovery day between performances so your voice has time to heal before using it again

Let's break down that bullshit!

First of all, "saving your voice" is impossible. The concept of saving your voice is like asking the doctor to put a cast on your leg to prevent you from breaking it. Putting a cast on your leg before you've broken it does nothing useful because the cast is how you repair a break that has already occurred, NOT how you prevent a break from happening. Likewise, putting yourself on vocal rest before you damage your voice does absolutely nothing because vocal rest is how you repair vocal damage, NOT how you prevent it.

But the problem goes deeper than that. When you decide to be completely silent all day in an attempt to "save your voice" for a big gig that night, you actually put your voice in serious danger! Asking the voice to perform difficult vocal gymnastics after a period of complete silence is a fast way to cause vocal damage. The voice needs to be warm and active to perform big singing without causing potential problems.

The same concept is true for dancers, which is why you frequently see them dressed in multiple layers of clothing stretching periodically through the day. A dancer who has a principal dance role in a musical or a ballet can't spend the day lounging on the couch and then go straight into her performance without risking injury. Muscles that aren't warmed up have a difficult time performing optimally, especially if the required task is intense.

So, giving your voice muscles the day off when you plan to ask a lot of them that night will have the opposite effect of what you desire. Even proper vocal rest isn't complete silence. You need do some light humming three to four times each day to keep the voice active and warm during a rest period.

Secondly, as for all the "healing" treatments, please remember, THERE ARE NO QUICK FIXES FOR VOCAL DAMAGE. Your teas, lozenges, throat sprays, medicines, and elixirs, may be all-natural, healthy, organic, and non-toxic, but they are NOT SOLUTIONS for voice loss. No matter what the marketing or the glowing recommendations from your best friend might be, these treatments can only supplement good technique. And if you implement proper technique, you'll have no need for these supplements.

They may not be "dangerous" on their own, but if you choose to put your trust in them to fix your vocal damage problem, you create a risky situation. Most of these kinds of "solutions" will dull the senses or numb the pain so you no longer feel it. But pain is an indication that there's a problem. If you suddenly are pain-free, you're going to feel bold enough to make different decisions with your voice. Once the effects of the "solution" wear off, you'll be left with more pain than you felt before taking it. You could cause serious damage to your voice because you can't feel the pain of your actions until it's too late.

Lastly, believing you need a day to recover between gigs is a fast path to being unable to earn enough income, having to turn down work, and perpetuating the myth that voice loss will inevitably happen to you. Schedule time off for yourself because you WANT it, not because your voice needs time to recover. If you follow the steps laid out in this book, you won't NEED a recovery day.

If you'd like to work with me on achieving Unlimited Vocal Health for yourself, let's have a chat about what it would look like for you:

www.getmypowerup.com

THIS IS THE END; HOLD YOUR BREATH AND COUNT TO TEN

> "At the end of the road is the beginning of a new adventure."
> – Unknown

It's that time. I hope very much to have opened your eyes to see what's possible for you – to see opportunity instead of limitation. The only way to change the belief system of the performance industry about vocal health is to stop the spread of the myths, lies, and bad information and to educate as many performers and coaches as possible about the truth. Voice loss and vocal fatigue are NOT inevitable. They are PREVENTABLE.

I've shown you how to prevent vocal issues from occurring in your life, but it's completely understandable to have questions or want feedback on your efforts as you implement what you've read. You won't find any other coach who teaches this method. You may find coaches who teach pieces of it along with some other bullshit. You'll need discernment to weed it out.

I don't want you to go back to your old habits, lies, and myths of what you believed before reading this book. You deserve to have a voice that is available for you ALL the time, one that can do more than you ever thought possible. When you're ready to take the next step, one of my favorite ways to work with clients is inside my No Limits Academy, and I'd love to invite you to join it.

The No Limits Academy is a place where my clients gain seemingly superhuman performance abilities that lead to achieving incredible results. Every month, we meet to learn a new skill and receive a challenge for implementing the skill into our day-to-day lives. At the end of the month, everyone in the class gets one-on-one time with me in front of the group to work on anything for my feedback and critique. The best part about these end-of-the-month classes is that you learn from your own time in the hot seat, as well as from observing the coaching your classmates receive.

In between those two monthly classes, there is an active online community where members have the opportunity to upload videos each week of their practice for my feedback and critique. As a bonus, members get access to my entire library of training videos for a whole year so they can learn anything they need related to performance from a reliable and healthy source right at their fingertips. The Academy is like having an on-demand vocal coach in your back pocket at all times. No matter what topic we cover in the Academy, you have the ability to get feedback, answers, and critique on whatever you are working on – inside or outside of the contents contained in this book.

If you resonate with what you read in this book but need a little help with implementing it, the No Limits Academy is the place to be. It's the best place to go for accountability on keeping your vocal health practice active in your life.

To join the Academy, visit this link on the Sing Without Limits website:

www.singwithoutlimits.com/membership/no-limits-academy-membership

I look forward to partnering with you as you begin your adventure into Unlimited Vocal Health™

THANK YOU FOR BEING A FRIEND

"As we express our gratitude, we must never forget that the highest appreciation is not to utter words, but to live by them."

– John F. Kennedy

I have so many people to thank for helping me develop this method and write this book. For starters, I'd like to thank my voice teachers – Mrs. Mueller, Cynthia, and Bill – for giving me a solid foundation, for encouraging me to continue, and for giving me the opportunity to completely understand and discover technique.

I also want to thank my clients for their willingness to put their faith in me with their voices. It's because of them that I'm able to have proof and confidence in my method.

I want to thank my author coach Vickie Gould, for her brilliance and encouragement and for helping me write two books in one year.

I must thank my superstar assistant Chloe, for her hours of hard work that she does so excellently, for being my support when I need it, and for her creative genius in everything she does, including the book covers for both of my books.

Thank you to Jeanne, Bryce, Tucker, and Dora; to Glyenis, Alex, Cody, and Ashley; to Nanci, Jack, Alfie, and Ziggy, and of course James, for a fantastic environment for writing. Thank you also James, for your endless support and encouragement.

Thank you to the McGhee Law Firm and Trademark My Stuff for your services in helping me acquire my trademark. Thanks also to Mark Goodman, Esq., for your services in helping me acquire my patent.

Thank you to my mom who paid for all my voice lessons and education, who supported every crazy dream I've had, and who continues to encourage me in everything I do. I don't even know who I'd be without you.

Thank you in advance to the first major recording artist who puts your trust in me to help you never lose your voice again. I know I can help you, and I thank you in advance for giving me the chance to change your singing career for good.

IF THEY ASKED ME, I COULD WRITE A BOOK

"Every secret of a writer's soul, every experience of his life, every quality of his mind, is written large in his works."

– Virginia Woolf

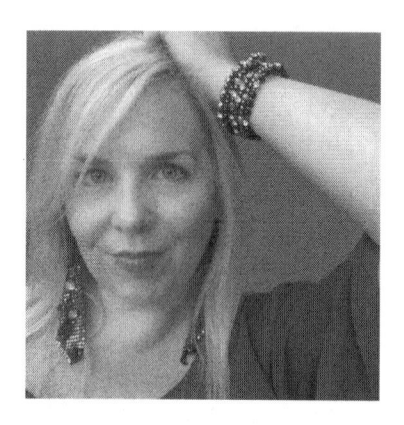

Katti Power is a two-time world champion vocal coach, vocal health expert, speaker, and author of the international bestselling book, *Turns Out I'm HOT After All: How I Got My POWER Back After a Breakup (and how you can, too, no matter what's happened in your life)*. She helps singers, actors, and speakers book roles and gigs, win competitions, overcome stage fright, and find a unique style that's all their own, all without ever experiencing voice loss. She's also the Founder of the POWER Academy of Master Coaches where she trains and certifies vocal coaches to teach her vocal method to clients of their own. She has been a sought-after judge for regional, national, and international talent competitions. She does the bulk of her coaching online from her home in Las Vegas, NV.

Katti is the mommy to Marmalade, her sweet rescue kitty, who waited very impatiently for this book to be written so she could have some lovins.

When she's not coaching, writing, judging competitions, or rubbing Marmalade's belly, she can be found in her favorite place - the kitchen - creating authentic Italian dishes from scratch. She longs to visit Italy to study cooking with nonnas on the Amalfi Coast.

Learn more at **www.singwithoutlimits.com** and at **www.kattipower.com**.

Printed in Poland
by Amazon Fulfillment
Poland Sp. z o.o., Wrocław